The Neuroscience of Why Football Moves Us

When the Ball Moves

Football and the Hidden Life of the Game

Moawiah Naffaa

Copyright

When the Ball Moves
Football and the Hidden Life of the Game

This book explores human attention, emotion, memory, identity, behavior, and related aspects of brain function through the experience of football.

First edition, 2026

Published by Moawiah Naffaa

Author: Moawiah Naffaa
Email: **Moawiah.Naffaa@proton.me**

For everyone who first felt it as a child and never quite stopped feeling it

The ball moves across the field,

but the real movement happens inside us

The ball rolls across wet concrete.

Night settles over a small neighborhood field.
Floodlights hum above the pitch.
Someone shouts a name from the edge of the touchline.

A pass skips between two players.
Another runner cuts suddenly into space.

Before the ball reaches him, someone watching already senses where the move might go.

Attention narrows.
A body leans forward.
For an instant, the next moment seems to exist before it has happened.

The ball finds him.

One touch forward.
A shot.

The net snaps.

Voices break open into the night.

What happened on the field lasted only seconds. Somewhere else, breathing changed. Muscles tightened and released. A moment that had not existed a heartbeat earlier suddenly carried enough emotion to remain in memory for years.

For a brief instant, the entire world seems to narrow to the movement of a single ball.

Only later do we realize that the ball was never the only thing moving.

Table of Contents

PROLOGUE

When the Ball Moves

The ball is perfectly still.

That may be the strangest part.

A player stands a few steps behind it. Across from him, the goalkeeper waits on the line, knees slightly bent, trying to appear larger than the space he occupies.

Around them, the stadium is nearly motionless.

Beyond the stadium, the same moment is unfolding in living rooms, cafés, bars, airports, restaurants, hotel rooms, and public squares. People who have never met one another are staring at the same patch of grass.

Some are standing.

Some cannot look.

Some clasp their hands together.

Someone rises from a chair and sits back down.

A child watches the adults instead of the screen.

Millions of people are waiting for one person to kick one stationary ball.

And their bodies are already reacting.

Breathing changes.

Shoulders tighten.

Eyes narrow.

Conversations stop.

The referee blows the whistle.

The player begins to move.

Before his foot reaches the ball, the goalkeeper has already started making a prediction.

So has everyone watching.

Left.
Right.
High.
Low.
Score.
Save.

For the briefest moment, several futures exist at once.

Then the foot strikes the ball.

Everything collapses into one.

This is football stripped to its simplest form: one player, one goalkeeper, one ball.

Yet the physical simplicity of the moment creates extraordinary complexity everywhere else.

Why should movement happening far away alter the breathing of someone sitting on a sofa?

Why do people lean when the ball bends toward the corner of the goal?

Why can a stranger's mistake ruin an evening?

Why can another stranger's goal send people running into streets?

Why can one second remain vivid for decades?

And why do we willingly return to this uncertainty again and again?

A football match takes place inside white lines, under known rules, within a fixed amount of time.

But the experience does not remain there.

It reaches attention.

Prediction.
The body.
Memory.
Identity.

Watch a dangerous attack begin.

A midfielder turns.

A runner accelerates into space.

The pass has not been played yet, but people are already moving in their seats.

For a moment, everyone is waiting for something that does not yet exist.

The game keeps asking the same quiet question:

What happens next?

We rarely notice how quickly we answer.

A defender steps forward and danger seems closer.

Half a meter opens on the wing, and expectation rises.

A goalkeeper shifts his weight and an entire room reacts.

The body begins participating before the outcome is known.

Then something even stranger happens.

A goal crosses the line and people who would have passed one another silently in the street suddenly grab each other by the shoulders. Thousands of separate reactions become one roar.

Football makes emotion public.

It also begins earlier than we usually realize.

A child can know that a match matters before knowing why.

The child sees adults become quiet, watches someone lean toward the television, hears a voice rise, and feels the room change.

The rules can come later.

The feeling is already there.

Years pass, and a strange word appears.

We.

We scored.

We lost.

We are going through.

The players may never know the supporter's name. The club may be thousands of miles away. Yet somehow the pronoun changes.

The contradiction is a clue.

So is what happens after the final whistle.

The match stops.

The mind sometimes does not.

After disappointment, another fixture eventually appears, carrying a new date and a new possibility.

Years after I first learned to love football, studying the brain changed the questions I asked while watching it.

I began noticing things that once seemed too ordinary to deserve attention.

A supporter leaning before the pass arrived.

Thousands recognizing danger almost together.

A single football memory remaining vivid while whole seasons around it faded.

The football had not changed.

The questions had.

What looked like a game also began to reveal attention, prediction, identity, memory, and shared emotion unfolding in real time.

They were parts of one lived experience.

The brain does not experience these things separately. Prediction can change the body, emotion can change memory, identity can change perception, and other people can change the intensity of all of them.

The ball rests on the penalty spot.

The goalkeeper waits.

The player begins his run.

Somewhere far away, someone who cannot influence any of it stops breathing for a second.

The remarkable thing is not only where the ball goes.

It is what happens everywhere else when it moves.

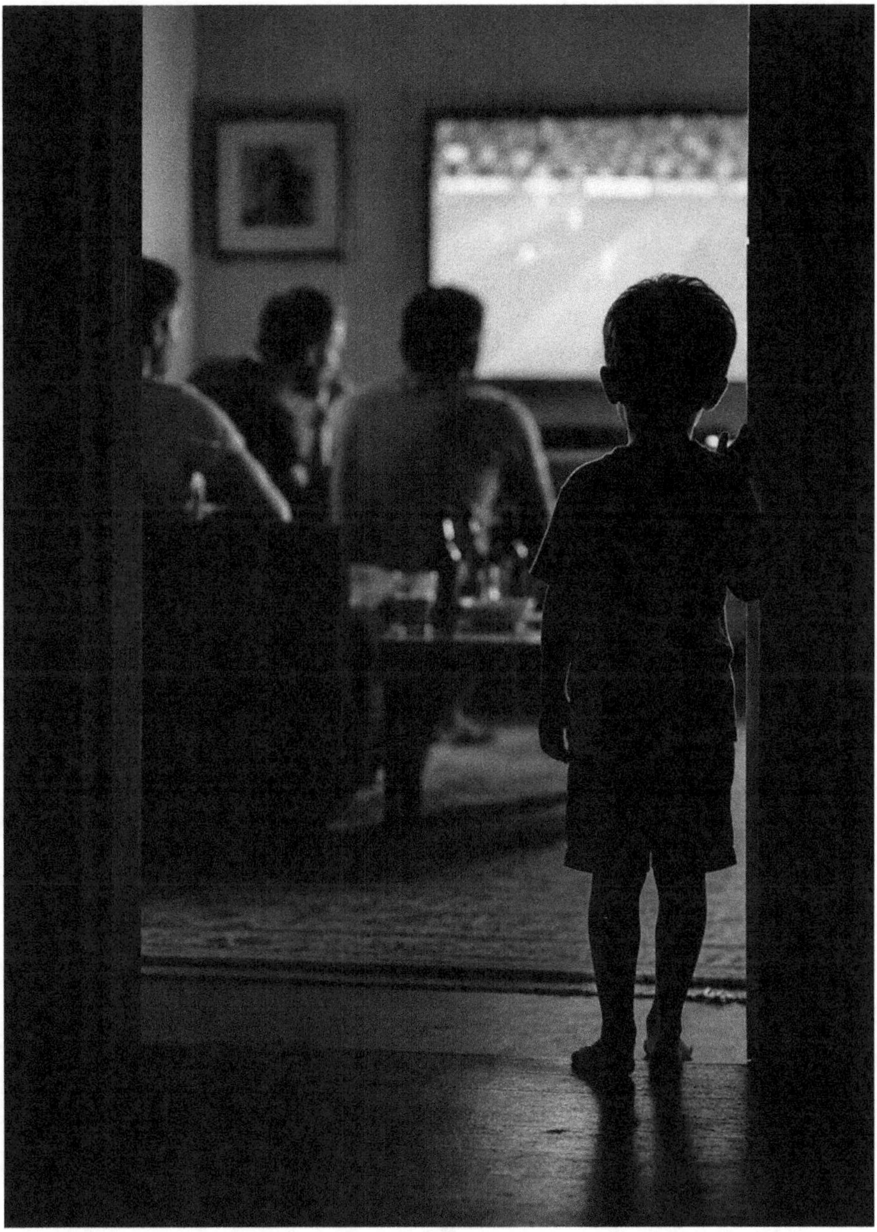

PART I — BEFORE THE WHISTLE

How Football Enters Us Before the Match Begins

Football often enters a life before anyone decides to let it in.

It may begin with a sound from another room. A crowd rising through a television. A voice suddenly sharper than it was a moment before. A silence that makes a child look up.

Before tactics, there is atmosphere.

Before allegiance, there are other people caring.

Before anyone understands formations, competitions, or why one goal matters more than another, there is the unmistakable feeling that something important is happening.

A child notices.

Someone shifts toward the screen.
Someone becomes quiet.
Someone shouts.

The room changes.

At first, the emotion belongs to everyone else. The child is watching the people as much as the match, learning from faces, voices, gestures, and the sudden changes in energy that move through the room.

Understanding comes later.

Attachment rarely begins with a formal decision. It grows through repetition: a sound heard often enough, a color that becomes recognizable, a name spoken with feeling, a game that keeps returning to the life around you.

Little by little, what once belonged to other people starts to acquire personal weight.

The distant team on the screen feels closer. Results begin to feel consequential. Colors become recognizable. Names acquire history.

Then language shifts.

We.

The word can arrive so naturally that no one notices the moment it happens.

What was once happening to a group of strangers somewhere else has crossed an invisible boundary. The game is no longer entirely outside the person watching it.

Once that boundary has moved, the game begins to matter even when it is not being played.

The match does not need to be underway for attention to drift toward it. A coming fixture can already occupy part of the day. The future has not arrived, yet it has begun to matter.

First, we feel something without fully understanding it.

Then we recognize ourselves inside it.

Eventually, we find ourselves waiting for what has not happened yet.

The attachment is there.

The identity is there.

The expectation is there.

The match has not begun.

But we have already entered it.

CHAPTER 1 — BEFORE WE UNDERSTAND

Some of my earliest memories of football are not really memories of football.

They are memories of sound.

A crowd rising through a television.

Voices changing somewhere nearby.

The sudden sharpness of an adult reaction.

A few seconds of tension followed by noise.

I could not have explained the structure of the game, the logic of a formation, or why one match mattered more than another.

But I knew that it mattered.

That came first.

A child does not need a tactical vocabulary to recognize importance.

Faces change.

Voices rise.

Conversation disappears for a few seconds.

Then something happens on the screen and the atmosphere shifts again.

The event itself may still be unclear. The emotional difference is much easier to read.

Something good happened.

Something bad happened.

Something nearly happened.

Children are constantly learning from changes like these. They notice expressions, tone, movement, tension, laughter, frustration, and relief. Other people reveal what deserves attention long before anyone deliberately explains why.

Football is especially generous with such signals.

A goal does not produce the same response as a harmless pass across midfield. A missed penalty changes the sound of a room. A late chance can pull everyone toward the same moment at once.

For a child still learning the game, those differences carry information.

Certain colors acquire significance.

A player's name sounds different because of the way adults say it.

A familiar song is attached to excitement.

A match carries an atmosphere unlike the programs around it.

Feeling can precede understanding.

We often imagine attachment forming in the opposite direction: first understanding the game, then deciding whether to care about it.

Football can arrive earlier.

The rules may still be incomplete while associations are already taking shape.

A child repeatedly encounters excitement attached to particular teams, colors, names, and moments. One match follows another, bringing recognizable voices and emotional rhythms with it.

Familiarity accumulates.

Soon, a team is no longer merely one set of shirts among many. A name no longer sounds interchangeable with every other name. Some moments draw attention more quickly than others.

Repetition has given them weight.

At first, much of the emotion is borrowed from the people nearby.

A dangerous attack develops and the adults tense.

The child tenses too.

A shot goes in and everyone celebrates.

The child joins them.

Borrowed emotion is one way human beings learn where attention belongs.

A child crossing a street learns something from the adult who stops at the curb, looks both ways, and reaches for a hand. The adult's behavior already marks the situation as important.

Football draws on the same social-learning pattern.

An adult shifts forward as play approaches the penalty area. Silence settles before a penalty. A goal releases the tension at once. A missed chance leaves disappointment behind.

The pattern is visible without explanation.

Repeated often enough, it starts to work from the inside.

The developing brain is constantly learning what deserves attention. Other people help mark the world before a child can explain it. A change in voice, posture, or expression can give an ordinary event emotional weight. Repeated pairings gradually transfer that weight to the event itself. The crowd rises often enough, the same colors return, the same names arrive with feeling, and eventually the signals no longer need an interpreter.

The child no longer has to wait for everyone else.

A pass opens space, and attention sharpens.

A player approaches goal, and the moment already feels different.

A shot leaves the foot, and the outcome matters before anyone nearby has responded.

The game itself now produces the feeling.

Understanding catches up gradually.

The lines on the field gain purpose. Attack and defense become easier to recognize. Certain players stand out. The logic of competition grows clearer.

Much of the emotional groundwork is already there.

The child is learning the rules of something that has been carrying feeling for a long time.

Early football memories are often strangely incomplete.

The score may disappear while the atmosphere survives.

A voice can remain clearer than a lineup. A particular light, a shirt, the glow of a television, or a sudden burst of noise can outlast the details of the match itself.

Emotion and attention help determine what stays.

For a child, the people surrounding a match can become part of the memory of the match.

Years later, the sequence of play may be gone while the feeling remains intact.

Attachment does not need a single dramatic beginning.

It can gather quietly across ordinary moments: a match watched here, a name heard again, a conversation overheard, an emotion copied before its cause was fully known.

Eventually, the child who once watched other people watching football starts watching the football itself.

The shift is easy to miss.

No ceremony marks it.

Nobody announces that the game has crossed from the room into the person.

But something has changed.

Questions appear.

Who are we playing?

Did we win?

When are they playing again?

The vocabulary is simple.

The emotional position is not.

Attention that once followed other people's responses now belongs to the game itself.

What began as borrowed excitement now generates excitement of its own.

The child no longer needs someone else to look worried before sensing danger.

No one has to celebrate first.

No one has to explain that the result matters.

The team on the screen is still made up of strangers. The child has not trained with them, traveled with them, or stepped onto the field beside them.

Yet the distance has started to shrink.

Soon, a small word will reveal just how far.

We.

CHAPTER 2 — THE MOMENT WE SAY "WE"

We scored.

It is an ordinary sentence in football.

It is also a strange one.

The supporter did not touch the ball.

Did not make the run.

Did not train all week.

Did not receive instructions in the dressing room.

May be sitting in another city, another country, or on another continent.

And yet when the ball crosses the line, the sentence comes naturally.

We scored.

Not they.

We.

That small word reveals how far attachment can travel.

A team starts as something outside us. Eleven players step onto a field wearing particular colors, carrying a particular name, playing beneath a badge that may have existed long before any current supporter was born.

At first, these things can be little more than information.

Then they acquire weight.

The colors become recognizable.

The badge grows familiar.

Certain names stay with us.

Past victories are retold.

Old defeats remain difficult to forget.

A history we never personally lived can still feel inherited.

The team no longer feels like a collection of strangers. It carries a place inside the supporter's sense of self.

Human beings do this far beyond football.

We attach ourselves to families, cities, schools, professions, communities, nations, traditions, and ideas. Membership changes the way events reach us.

A city we call home is praised, and the praise feels warmer.

A group we identify with succeeds, and some part of the success seems to travel back toward us.

Belonging changes emotional ownership.

Belonging also changes what the mind treats as personally relevant. The brain does not respond only to what happened; it responds to what the event is connected to. Once a team has been drawn into the self, its outcomes arrive carrying some of the weight normally reserved for things much closer to us. The goal is still scored by someone else. The emotional consequence no longer feels entirely external.

Football makes that change easy to hear.

It appears in the pronouns.

We won.

We lost.

We need a goal.

We cannot defend like this.

The language places the supporter inside an event being performed by other people.

The supporter remains outside the field.

Emotionally, the distance is smaller.

A neutral match can be beautiful without carrying much personal consequence. A supporter may admire the passing, the movement, the skill, the precision.

Put one of those teams inside the supporter's sense of identity, and the same kinds of passes, tackles, mistakes, and goals feel different.

A missed chance frustrates.

A late equalizer brings relief.

A victory can brighten an evening.

A defeat can follow someone home.

The event has acquired personal relevance without becoming a personal action.

The supporter is not the player. The supporter is invested in the player's fate.

Attachment does not depend on proximity. A child may discover a club on television, inherit it from family across countries, or follow a player first and stay after the player leaves.

Sometimes the connection is local. The stadium sits nearby, the streets change on match day, and the club feels woven into the city.

Sometimes it grows from one remarkable match, one tournament, one player, or one period of life in which the team happened to be present.

The origin varies.

The symbols remain.

A shirt is fabric.

Until it is not.

A badge is a design.

Until it carries memories.

A color is a wavelength of light.

Until one version of it appears in a stadium and thousands of people rise.

Objects acquire significance because people repeatedly place memory, loyalty, and experience inside them.

Put on the shirt and the body has not changed.

The social position has.

An affiliation is now visible.

A stranger wearing the same colors can suddenly feel less strange.

Two supporters may meet in an airport thousands of miles from the club they follow and begin talking as if part of the introduction has already happened.

The badge is enough to open the conversation.

A manager's name, a famous goal, a painful defeat, a season neither has forgotten—shared history fills the rest.

The relationship may last five minutes.

Recognition can arrive in seconds.

A chant reveals the same principle in another form.

One voice alone is small.

Thousands singing the same words produce something different.

The individual voice joins something larger.

For a while, the self sits inside a wider identity.

That widened identity is audible in the language supporters use.

Someone watching from a sofa can say:

We have to recover before Saturday.

The supporter will not attend training.

The sentence is still perfectly natural.

Its grammar does not describe physical contribution.

It describes identification.

The team's fate has been pulled close enough to the self that ordinary language treats the two as connected.

That connection becomes especially clear when the result is uncertain.

A neutral match can offer suspense.

With an attached team, the uncertainty carries personal stakes.

Every attack threatens something that matters.

Every defensive mistake feels heavier.

The final minutes stretch.

Relief sharpens.

The scoreboard is no longer emotionally neutral.

One number belongs to us.

The other belongs to them.

Every **we** creates a boundary.

Inside that boundary are shared memory, shared symbols, shared expectation, and shared joy.

A supporter can enter a stadium among tens of thousands of strangers and feel surrounded by people who want the same outcome.

The same connection can exist in a café, a family home, a small bar, or across messages sent between different countries.

The people involved may have little else in common.

For the duration of the match, one result matters to all of them.

Victory often feels larger in company because others carry the feeling with us. That identity can make defeat feel collective.

The result belongs to the team.

The feeling belongs to everyone who has made the team part of themselves.

A child who once asked what was happening eventually asks a different question.

Are we winning?

The distance between the screen and the self has narrowed.

The players are still strangers.

The badge is still a symbol.

The ball is still moving somewhere else.

But the outcome no longer belongs entirely to them.

It belongs, in some small emotional way, to us.

CHAPTER 3 — THE HOURS BEFORE KICKOFF

The match is still hours away.
Nothing has happened.
No pass has been misplaced.
No chance has been missed.
No referee has made a decision anyone can argue about.
The players may not even be at the stadium yet.
And still, the match has already entered the day.
You check the kickoff time.
You already know the kickoff time.
A few minutes later, you check it again.
Not because the hour has changed.
Because part of your attention has already moved toward the match.
The mind is occupied by an event that does not yet exist.
A future match can alter the present.

The morning feels different because of something scheduled for the evening. Ordinary tasks continue, but part of the mind keeps drifting elsewhere.
A conversation turns briefly toward who might start.
A phone is checked for team news.
One possible lineup appears.
Then another.
What if the manager changes formation?
What if the injured player is fit?
What if the new signing starts?
What if the opponent presses high?
What if we score first?
None of these events has happened.
Most never will.
But each one briefly creates a version of the match inside the mind.

The mind rarely waits passively for events. It estimates, prepares, imagines, and revises.

It is constantly leaning slightly ahead of the present. From incomplete information, it builds small models of what may happen next and begins organizing attention around them. Most disappear before we notice them. Others acquire enough emotional weight to change the present before the future has done anything at all.

Football gives that habit a clear target: one match, one opponent, one starting time.

Before the whistle, several outcomes can still be imagined.

It might be comfortable.

It might be tense.

It might turn on one moment no one forgets.

Before kickoff, all of them remain available.

Reality has not removed any of them yet.

That openness creates a peculiar kind of optimism.

Even supporters who know their team's weaknesses can construct a path to victory.

The defense has been poor lately, but perhaps today it holds.

The striker has not scored for weeks, but perhaps this is the day.

The opponent is stronger, but stronger teams lose.

A difficult season can recede from the imagination for a few hours because one match remains unwritten.

The future is generous before evidence begins narrowing it.

Waiting also develops its own rituals.

Someone chooses the shirt associated with an old victory and leaves another one in the drawer. Someone arrives at a familiar café earlier than necessary. Someone takes the usual place on the sofa and feels oddly reluctant to move.

These actions cannot choose the lineup, make the pass, or stop the opponent.

They give structure to the hours before kickoff.

A familiar action brings structure to a situation whose outcome remains uncontrollable.

That small sense of control can be comforting.

It turns waiting into preparation.

Superstition pushes the same impulse further.

The supporter knows that a shirt, seat, or café cannot affect the match, yet changing them can still feel wrong.

Emotion gives coincidence a long memory.
You wore that shirt when the team won.
You sat there during the comeback.
You watched from that café when everything went right.
The association can still acquire psychological force.
A pre-match ritual cannot control the ball.
It can change the experience of waiting for it to move.
Anticipation itself can be pleasurable.
Before kickoff, victory has not been earned.
It has not been lost either.
The desired outcome can still be imagined without contradiction from reality.
An event can affect us long before it occurs.

A holiday can lift the mood before departure. An important meeting can create tension hours before anyone enters the room.

Anticipation pulls the emotional consequences of an event into the present.
Football provides this experience with unusual regularity.

Fixtures appear on calendars days or weeks in advance. Supporters know what is coming, and the coming match creates a point toward which the week seems to lean.

There is Tuesday.
There is Wednesday.
There is Thursday.
And then there is Saturday.
The match organizes time before it occupies time.
As kickoff approaches, imagination has less room to wander.
The lineup is released.
The player expected to start is on the bench.
An injured defender is missing.
The formation is different.
A teenager has been selected unexpectedly.
What had been vague is suddenly more concrete.
Predictions adjust.
So does expectation.
Perhaps the change is good.
Perhaps the new formation will work.

Perhaps the player everyone doubted will have the match of his life.
The pre-match mind can turn surprisingly little information into a reason to believe.
Then kickoff approaches.
The freedom to imagine begins to narrow.
Once the ball moves, possibility meets evidence.
The opening minutes answer questions that had existed only in thought.
Is the team nervous?
Is the press working?
Is there space behind the defense?
Each answer closes one path and strengthens another.
The imagined match gives way to the one actually being played.
Before that moment, however, several versions can still coexist.

The match is not yet happening on the field, but it is already present in attention, expectation, conversation, and ritual.
A lineup.
A message.
A quiet confidence.
A fear of conceding early.
An image of the first goal.
Nothing has happened on the field.

Yet attention has shifted, predictions have formed, and the future has already entered the present.
The players walk toward the tunnel.
The clock approaches the hour.
Soon there will be only one version of the match.
For a little longer, there are many.
The match begins in the mind before it begins on the field.

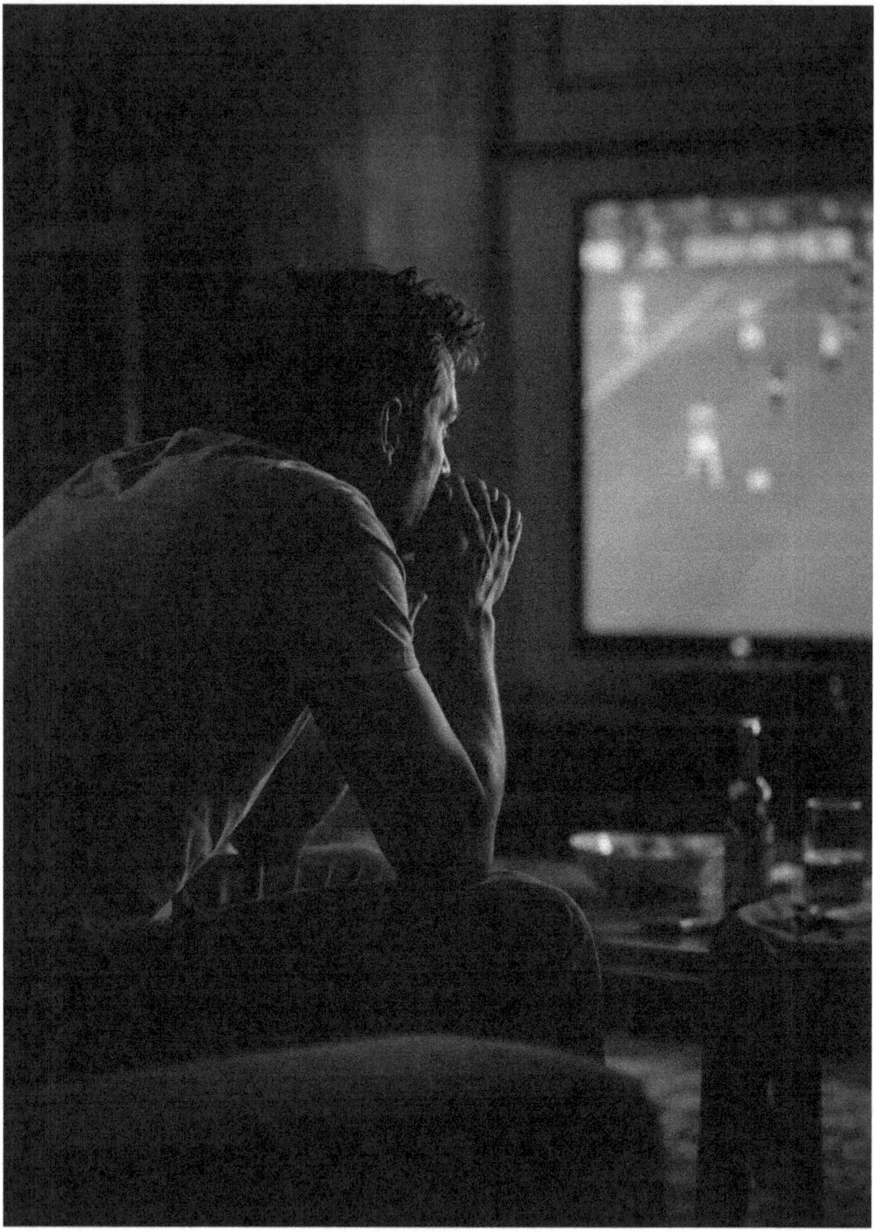

PART II — INSIDE THE MATCH

What Ninety Minutes Do to Attention, Body, Time, and Crowds

The whistle sounds.

Everything imagined before kickoff now meets the match itself.

Prediction meets evidence.
Confidence is tested.
Possibility begins narrowing into events that can no longer be taken back.

A pass succeeds.
Another fails.
Space opens and disappears.
A match that looked one way a minute ago begins to look different.

Watching from outside the field does not create emotional distance from what happens inside it.

The match keeps asking for attention because the next moment remains unsettled.

Ninety minutes will contain movement, waiting, uncertainty, release, and moments that seem to carry more weight than the clock gives them.

None of those experiences belongs entirely to the field.

The match is being played there.

It is being experienced somewhere else.

CHAPTER 4 — THE BODY THAT WILL NOT STAY STILL

The ball is played wide.

The winger reaches it before the defender and takes one touch toward the corner of the penalty area.

The cross begins to bend.

Someone watching from a sofa leans with it.

Not dramatically.

Perhaps only a few centimeters.

The head tilts. The shoulders shift. The torso follows the flight of the ball as though movement in the living room could somehow help carry it toward the right place.

No movement there can change the cross.

And yet the lean happens.

Seeing action is not the same as receiving information from a distance. The brain is continuously estimating direction, speed, intention, and what is likely to happen next. When movement unfolds quickly, perception is closely linked to systems that prepare action.

We do not watch movement with the eyes alone.

Imagine seeing a glass slip from someone's hand.

Before it reaches the floor, your hand may twitch or your shoulders tighten, even when you are too far away to catch it.

The response reflects the close relationship between perception and action.

Football makes that relationship unusually easy to see.

A defender slides into a tackle and a supporter's leg tightens. A striker shapes to shoot and someone rises halfway from a chair. A loose ball drops inside the penalty area and breath is held until someone reaches it.

These reactions may last only a fraction of a second.

They are still part of watching.

When we observe another person move, the nervous system represents aspects of what that person is doing: where the movement is going, what it may accomplish, how quickly it is unfolding, and what could follow.

For the player, that preparation can turn into action.

For the supporter, it appears in smaller traces: a tightened thigh, a forward shift, a hand gripping the edge of a seat, a sudden shout.

The preparation has nowhere useful to go.

It still changes the person watching.

Consider a counterattack.

The ball is recovered near midfield.

One player turns immediately.

Another is already running.

There are three defenders back.

Then two.

The passing lane opens.

The supporter sees it before the pass arrives.

The torso moves forward. The feet shift beneath the chair. Posture changes.

Prediction has already become physical.

The nervous system does not need a conscious instruction to begin preparing. Readiness can appear first in muscle tension, posture, breathing, and the tiny adjustments that precede deliberate movement. The supporter will never complete the action on the field. The body can still prepare for the direction the moment seems to be taking.

The pass is played.

Now the attack accelerates.

Attention narrows around the runner and the ball. Muscles tighten. Breathing changes. The spectator follows the developing move not only with vision but with a state of readiness.

Different moments organize that readiness differently.

Fast action can pull the body forward.

Danger can produce tension.

A decisive moment can produce stillness.

Watch a room just before a penalty.

People who were moving seconds earlier stop.

Hands remain where they are. Conversation disappears. Breathing becomes shallow.

The stillness is concentrated readiness.

Then the kick is taken.

The reaction can arrive before language does.

A dangerous pass is played.
The body shifts.
Then thought catches up.
The shout can come before the sentence.
The hands can reach the head before the explanation for the miss has been formed.

The nervous system is already tracking movement and estimating its consequences while conscious interpretation is still arriving.

A moment later come the words.
"He should have passed."
"The keeper moved early."
"I thought that was in."
By then, the physical response has already happened.
Football repeatedly creates these brief gaps between reaction and explanation.
A shot leaves the foot and someone rises.
The goalkeeper reaches it.
The danger ends.
Shoulders drop.
Air comes out.
The supporter sits again.
Preparation.
Suspension.
Release.
The sequence may last only seconds, but it can repeat throughout an entire match.
An attack develops and readiness rises.
The danger passes and tension falls.
Another attack begins.
The cycle returns.

That repeated movement between readiness and release helps explain why watching an intense match can feel physically tiring even when the supporter has barely left the seat.

Muscles have tightened and relaxed.
Breathing has changed.
Attention has repeatedly narrowed around danger.

The physical demands are modest, but the experience still recruits posture, breath, muscle tension, and attention.

Movement on the field is translated into movement in the observer.

Not copied exactly.

Translated.

The observed action enters systems involved in understanding and preparing movement.

The result is participation without control.

Preparation can also disappear as quickly as it appears.

The pass is intercepted.

The runner is offside.

The shot is blocked.

A state of readiness is built and cancelled, sometimes several times within the same attack.

The match therefore has a physical rhythm beneath the visible one.

Not the rhythm of sprinting, tackling, or shooting.

The quieter rhythm of watching.

A spectator can finish a match and say, "I did nothing," while the body tells a more complicated story.

For ninety minutes, posture shifted with danger. Muscles prepared for outcomes. Breath changed with the movement of the ball. Attention pulled the body toward events happening somewhere else.

The supporter never entered the field.

The field entered the supporter.

Watching football is physically more participatory than it appears.

CHAPTER 5 — THE BEAUTIFUL UNCERTAINTY

A match can change with one touch.

A team can control possession for twenty minutes and concede from one counterattack.

A defender can read the pass correctly and still watch a deflection send the ball somewhere else.

A team that looks finished can score once and suddenly look dangerous again.

Football rarely allows certainty to settle for long.

That instability is one of the game's great attractions.

We often think pleasure comes from getting what we want.

Sometimes it comes from not yet knowing whether we will get it.

The score is level.

Ten minutes remain.

One team attacks.

The other clears.

A runner finds space.

The pass is delayed.

The opening disappears.

Another attack forms.

Nothing has been decided.

The mind keeps trying to get ahead of the game.

Who will receive the ball?

Will the defender step forward?

Will the winger cross?

Will the striker shoot?

Will the goalkeeper come?

Prediction is woven into watching.

A developing attack invites a forecast before the outcome arrives.

The midfielder will pass wide.

The defender will clear.
The goalkeeper will collect the cross.
Then something else happens.
The midfielder turns inside.
The defender slips.
The goalkeeper spills the ball.
The expected sequence breaks.
The mind had prepared one version of the next moment and received another.
That mismatch sharpens the experience.

The brain is continuously comparing what it expected with what actually arrives. When the two agree, little correction is needed. When they separate, attention is pulled toward the difference. The defender was supposed to clear. He did not. The goalkeeper was supposed to hold the ball. He did not. For a moment, the future has to be rebuilt.

A predictable match would offer less to anticipate.
Football refuses to stay that simple.
The favorite can struggle.
The underdog can score first.
The dominant side can hit the post three times and still trail.
A goalkeeper can make save after save and then misjudge one cross.
The game remains alive because possibility remains alive.
An underdog makes this especially visible.
One team has the better players.
More possession.
More chances.
More control.
But the score remains close.
Another minute passes.
Then another.
The expected goal does not come.
Maybe they can hold on.
Maybe one counterattack will be enough.
Maybe the favorite is getting nervous.
A result can remain unlikely while feeling increasingly imaginable.
The underdog reaches the final twenty minutes.
Then the final ten.

A corner is won.

For a few seconds, the advantage built over an entire match matters less than one delivery into the penalty area.

The defender may clear it.

The striker may reach it.

The goalkeeper may claim it.

The ball may fall somewhere no one expected.

No answer has arrived yet.

Missed chances make the same mechanism painfully clear.

A striker runs through on goal.

The obvious future forms immediately.

Score.

The shot goes wide.

For an instant, the goal existed as expectation.

Then reality removed it.

A team under pressure breaks forward.

A player who has barely touched the ball finds space.

One pass changes the geometry of the field.

Suddenly the side that looked close to conceding has the best chance of the match.

The game repeatedly refuses to honor the forecast that seemed safest a few seconds earlier.

The 2022 World Cup final between Argentina and France pushed that instability to an extreme.

For long stretches, Argentina appeared to have taken control.

A two-goal lead gave the match a clear direction.

Then France scored twice in rapid succession.

The final opened again.

Argentina scored in extra time.

France equalized again.

Certainty repeatedly arrived and disappeared.

Each time one ending seemed close, the match produced another.

By the closing stages, almost every attack carried enormous weight because the result remained unresolved.

The same structure appears every week whenever a one-goal lead, an underdog, or one late chance keeps the contest unresolved.

There is pleasure inside that waiting.

Uncertainty can be pleasurable and uncomfortable at the same time.

A close match can produce tension, frustration, restlessness, even the desire for the answer to arrive.

But imagine knowing the final score before kickoff.

You could still appreciate a beautiful goal.

You could still admire technique.

You could still notice tactical decisions.

Something central would be missing.

The question **What happens next?** would already have an answer.

Much of sport's pull depends on the fact that it does not.

The supporter watches because the result has not yet been chosen.

Each new event can alter the estimate.

A defender hesitates.

A midfielder turns instead of passing.

A striker shoots when everyone expected the extra touch.

The mind adjusts.

Surprise enters when events depart from the pattern we had prepared.

Sometimes the correction is small.

Sometimes it reorganizes the entire contest.

That constant openness changes the value of reward.

A goal at 4–0 does not usually feel like a goal at 0–0 in the final minute.

The physical event may be similar.

Its meaning is not.

When the match is still undecided, one goal can transform everything around it.

The reward is amplified by what it resolves.

A save can preserve one path.

A goal can create another.

A miss can leave the question open.

That is why a scoreless match can sometimes feel more gripping than one full of goals.

The scoreboard alone does not determine intensity.

Possibility does.

A match can be 0–0 and feel dangerously alive because either side might score.

Another can be 4–0 and feel emotionally finished with half an hour still to play.

The players keep running.

The clock keeps moving.

But the uncertainty has largely disappeared.

Attention loosens.

Conversation returns.

The urgency falls.

The game continues, but the question pulling the spectator forward has weakened.

While the future remains unsettled, hope and fear can occupy the same few seconds.

A defender receives the ball under pressure.

A midfielder turns.

A runner accelerates.

The passing lane opens.

For a fraction of a second, several outcomes remain alive.

The pass may arrive.

The defender may intercept it.

The runner may be offside.

The goalkeeper may reach it first.

Then the ball is played.

One outcome becomes real.

The others vanish.

Prediction.

Outcome.

Revision.

Prediction again.

The beauty is not only in seeing what happens.

It is in knowing, until the moment arrives, that it could have happened differently.

Uncertainty is not merely tolerated in football.

It is one of the forces that makes attention so intense.

CHAPTER 6 — WHEN TIME STOPS

Most seconds disappear.

They pass, make room for the next one, and leave almost nothing behind.

Then football produces a second that refuses to behave like the others.

The striker is through.

The goalkeeper is coming.

The ball drops into the space between them.

Everything seems to slow.

The run.

The touch.

The angle.

The goalkeeper's movement.

For an instant, the match feels larger than the clock measuring it.

Then the moment is gone.

But sometimes it does not leave.

Years later, the details can still return with surprising clarity.

Where you were.

Who was beside you.

What the room looked like.

What you expected to happen.

What actually happened.

A football match unfolds inside ordinary time.

The clock moves forward at the same rate whether the ball is near the half-way line or flying toward goal in the final seconds.

Experience does not.

Five quiet minutes can disappear almost unnoticed.

One dangerous second can dominate everything around it.

Clock time measures duration.

The mind measures significance.

Attention is never distributed evenly across a match.

A harmless pass across midfield does not demand the same concentration as a penalty. A routine clearance does not occupy the mind like a final attack.

As the stakes rise, attention tightens.

Background details fall away.

The field seems to narrow.

One movement carries more weight than the ordinary seconds around it.

A late chance shows this clearly.

The match is nearly over.

One team needs a goal.

The ball is played forward.

A defender misses it.

A striker reaches the space behind him.

The goalkeeper comes out.

On the clock, the sequence may last only seconds.

Inside the experience, it can feel stretched.

The supporter sees the ball descend, the striker prepare, the goalkeeper close the angle.

There seems to be enough time to imagine several endings before one arrives.

He's through.

This is it.

Then the shot is taken.

The clock did not slow.

Attention changed.

More of it was packed into those seconds, and concentrated attention can make experience feel denser.

Football produces this distortion again in a different form before a penalty.

The taker walks toward the ball.

The referee waits.

The goalkeeper moves along the line.

A few seconds can feel strangely long because almost everything else has dropped away.

The future of the moment seems concentrated into one action.

What happens during these episodes also affects what remains afterward.

We do not carry every minute of every match forward equally.

Entire stretches vanish.

Possession sequences blur together.

Routine substitutions disappear.

Even matches we remember loving can lose most of their detail.

What remains are often the moments that carried the greatest emotional weight.

The goal.

The miss.

The save.

The whistle.

The instant when the expected future changed.

A supporter may forget most of a season played ten years ago and still describe one shot from that same season with remarkable precision.

The surrounding weeks have faded.

The second remains.

Memory is selective.

Attention influences what enters strongly. Emotion gives some experiences greater weight. Later processes help stabilize certain traces more effectively than others.

The result is not a complete archive.

It is a landscape with peaks.

The brain does not preserve a match in proportion to how long each moment lasted. What received intense attention has an advantage. What arrived with surprise, fear, relief, or enormous consequence can leave a stronger trace than the ordinary minutes around it. A second does not need to last longer to occupy more memory.

Some moments rise far above everything around them.

Late in the 2022 World Cup final between Argentina and France, Randal Kolo Muani broke through toward goal.

Emiliano Martínez came out to meet him.

The shot arrived.

Martínez stopped it.

The sequence lasted only seconds, but the stakes concentrated extraordinary meaning into them.

One successful finish could have decided the final.

The save preserved another ending.

Brief action, concentrated attention, and enormous consequence give the moment unusual weight in memory.

A supporter may retain the angle of the run, Martínez spreading himself, and the instant the shot was blocked while much of the surrounding play fades.

The second occupies more memory than its duration on the clock would ever suggest.

A late winner can do the same.

So can a decisive miss.

The ball crosses the line, or fails to.

A single event can divide the match into before and after.

The clock records continuity.

Memory often records rupture.

Football is often remembered through moments rather than complete sequences.

The goal went in.

The penalty was missed.

The goalkeeper made the save.

Years later, the natural questions are often simple.

Where were you?

Who were you with?

Emotional memory often carries some of its surroundings with it. A goal can remain tied to a room, a café, a voice, or the light outside a window. Years later, one cue may bring the event back.

The memory itself is not a perfect recording. Details can fade, shift, or be reconstructed even when the central moment remains vivid.

What survives is often the emotional shape of the event.

The anticipation.

The action.

The realization that everything had changed.

A late winner may occupy only the final instant of a match, yet years later it can stand in for the entire night.

Mention the game and the mind may return immediately to that second.

Not the first throw-in.

Not the uneventful possession in midfield.

Not the long stretch in which little happened.

The decisive moment.

The rest of the match can look, in retrospect, like the road leading toward it.

Years pass. Players retire. Competitions move on.

The moment can still feel close.

One image may be enough.

The ball dropping.

The striker reaching it.

The goalkeeper spreading himself.

The shot.

The save.

Time passes evenly.

Experience does not.

Memory does not.

Some seconds barely register.

Others become landmarks.

And occasionally, one second grows large enough to outlive entire years around it.

CHAPTER 7 — THE EXPLOSION

A goal is scored.

For a fraction of a second, nothing seems organized.

A man throws both arms upward.

Someone behind him shouts before any words form.

Two strangers collide in an embrace.

A child jumps onto a chair.

A scarf disappears into the air.

Several rows of people surge forward.

The sound rises almost at once.

What began as thousands of separate reactions suddenly feels like one event.

The goal happened on the field.

The explosion happened everywhere else.

Football is full of individual emotion, but some of its most powerful moments are difficult to understand one person at a time.

A supporter can feel joy alone.

Put that same supporter among thousands of people waiting for one outcome, and the experience changes.

The people around us are not merely present.

They shape the emotion itself.

The nervous system is continuously reading the people around it. Faces, voices, posture, movement, and sound all become part of the emotional environment. One person's reaction therefore becomes information for another. The goal begins the response, but the crowd keeps feeding the response back into itself.

Before the goal, attention has already narrowed toward one patch of play.

A winger reaches the byline.

Heads turn together.

The cross is delivered.

Bodies rise.

The ball travels through the penalty area.

For those few seconds, thousands of people are tracking one object, anticipating one possibility, waiting for one answer.

Their attention has converged.

Then the header reaches the net.

The waiting ends everywhere at once.

If one supporter realized a goal had been scored ten seconds after everyone else, the reaction would feel different.

Part of the force comes from simultaneity.

The event reaches many people at nearly the same instant.

Faces change together.

Posture changes together.

Voices rise together.

One reaction becomes visible to another.

Then another.

Emotion moves through the group.

A supporter who might have smiled alone can shout in a crowd.

Someone who would have raised one hand at home may find both arms around a stranger.

The behavior of other people supplies information about the scale of the moment.

Their excitement confirms your own.

Your reaction confirms theirs.

The feeling gains volume.

Human beings are deeply responsive to one another.

A laugh can make another laugh easier.

Applause gathers strength when more people join it.

Football places these ordinary social tendencies inside moments of unusually concentrated attention.

Everyone is already looking in the same direction.

Everyone already cares about the immediate outcome.

Everyone receives the answer at almost the same instant.

The conditions for emotional coordination are already in place.

No one instructs strangers when to throw their arms around one another.

No central voice says: now shout.

Yet thousands of bodies can produce something remarkably ordered.

A chant gives a clearer version of the same process.

One voice starts.

A few nearby voices join.

The words spread.

Soon an entire stand is singing at the same tempo.

People who arrived separately are now breathing between the same lines, producing the same words, following one rhythm.

The individual voice is still there.

It has joined something larger.

Rhythm makes coordination easier.

A repeated chant gives people a structure: a familiar phrase, a predictable beat, a clear moment to enter.

Once enough voices join, the chant acquires mass.

Someone who was silent hears the people around them and joins.

The sound grows.

More voices enter.

Movement can organize in the same way.

A stand rises. Scarves lift. Hands clap in rhythm. Bodies bounce together.

None of these actions changes the score.

They change the social experience of it.

The football on the field may be identical to the football seen from a sofa.

The emotional environment is not.

At home, a goal may produce joy.

Inside a stadium, the same goal arrives surrounded by voices, bodies, gestures, and faces already responding.

Emotion is surrounded by evidence of itself.

Joy is seen, heard, felt in the movement nearby, and returned.

Collective emotion does not always arrive as noise.

A dangerous free kick is awarded.

Conversation drops.

People stand.

The taker places the ball.

Then comes another form of coordination.

Silence.

Thousands of people become quiet around one uncertainty.

The silence is not empty.

It is shared attention.

The whistle goes.

The ball rises.

For an instant, everyone waits.

The shot clears the wall and bends wide.

Sound rushes back.

Relief, frustration, groans, applause, voices.

The group has moved through the same transition around the same event.

A smaller room can produce its own version.

A crowded café watches a penalty.

Conversation disappears.

The kick is taken.

Goal.

The room erupts.

Someone who arrived alone is suddenly shouting with people whose names they do not know.

The event has supplied a temporary bond.

Shared attention can create social closeness with astonishing speed.

Two strangers may have little else in common and no expectation of ever meeting again.

For a few seconds, they wanted the same thing intensely.

Sometimes that is enough for a hug.

Football makes this kind of connection unusually easy because the emotional object is public.

The play is visible.

The score is understood.

The consequence is immediate.

No explanation is needed before the reaction begins.

A decisive goal can also escape the stadium almost instantly.

The ball crosses the line in one place.

Seconds later, windows open somewhere else.

A shout comes from an apartment.

A car horn answers from the street.

Phones begin ringing.

People spill from cafés.

Farther away, another room erupts.

A family may be watching in one country, friends in another, someone alone in a hotel room somewhere else.

The spaces are separate.

The emotional timing can still align.

Football creates temporary networks of attention.

For ninety minutes, people in different places organize parts of their lives around the same unfolding event.

Then one moment reaches all of them.

Distance weakens the physical feedback of a stadium, but shared timing can still connect separate rooms.

Messages arrive.

Calls begin.

The city sounds different.

The feeling travels through whatever channels are available.

Celebration reveals the amplification most clearly.

Joy invites expression, and expression invites response.

A raised arm is answered by another.

A chant gathers voices.

A stranger smiles and receives the same smile back.

The first reaction is to the football.

The next reactions are also to one another.

The feeling is still experienced individually, but its intensity is shaped by the people nearby.

They supply rhythm, confirmation, and energy.

A stadium acts like an emotional amplifier.

The goal supplies the spark; the people around it add force.

A person may embrace someone they would not normally touch.

Cry in front of people they would never otherwise meet.

Sing loudly despite rarely singing anywhere else.

For a few moments, ordinary social distance loosens because everyone understands what just happened.

Joy has a public language.

Raised arms.

A shout.

A hug.

A chant.

Sometimes tears.
The gestures are recognizable because others are doing them too.
Emotion finds form through the group.
Separate people acquire a temporary emotional center.
Attention points in one direction.
The answer arrives.
One reaction meets another.
Then another.
What began inside separate people grows through contact.
People do not merely experience emotion beside one another.
They amplify one another's emotion.

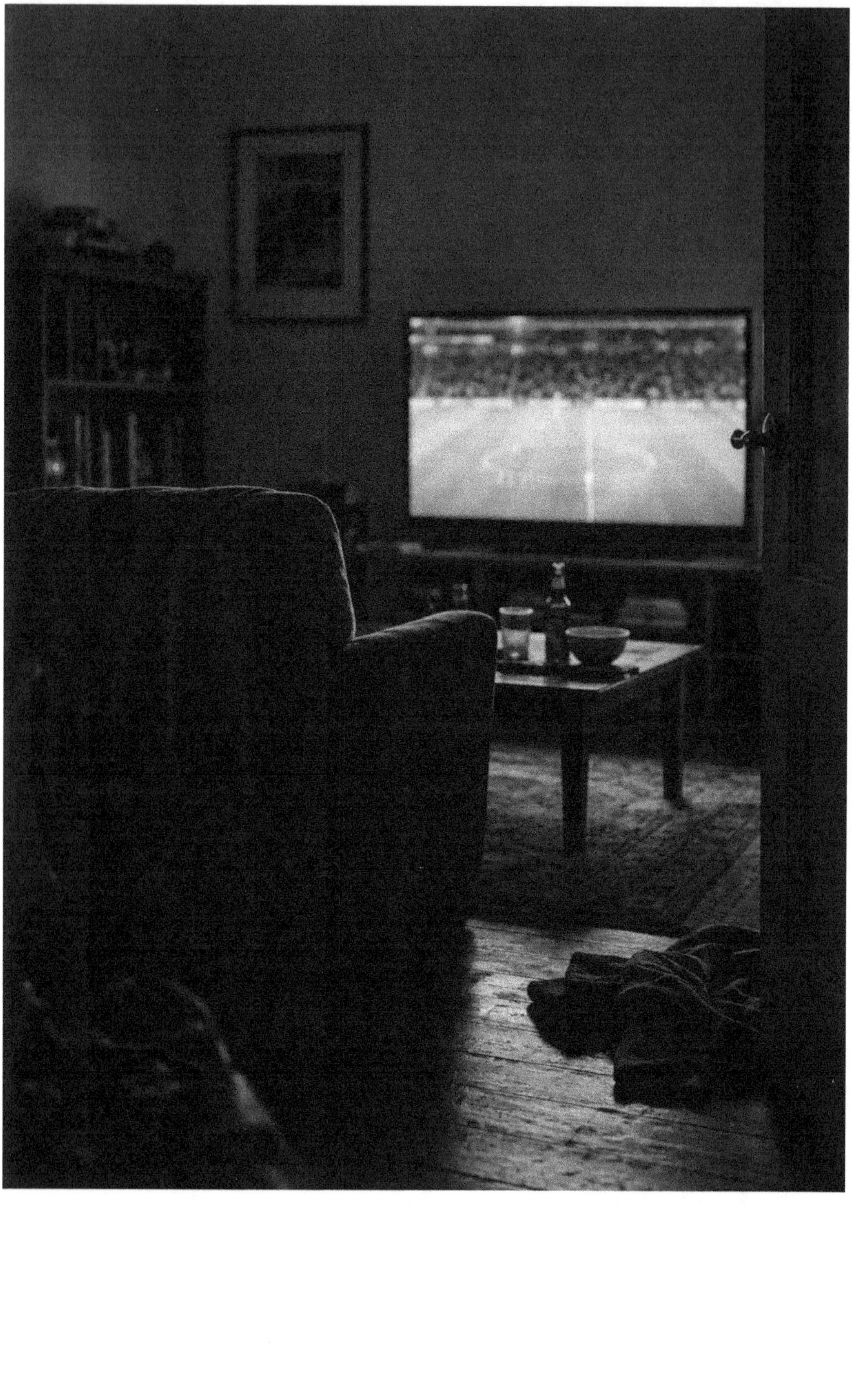

PART III — AFTER THE WHISTLE

Why Football Continues After Football Stops

The whistle blows.
The match is over.
The ball stops mattering almost immediately.
The score does not.
A few minutes earlier, everything was still moving toward an answer.
Now the answer exists.
One team has won.
One has lost.
The uncertainty has collapsed.
The stadium begins to empty.
Televisions are turned off.
People stand, gather their things, check their phones, look at one another.
Ordinary life starts returning.
But the match does not leave with the final whistle.
Sometimes disappointment settles slowly.
Sometimes it arrives all at once.
The game has ended, but the feeling does not disappear with it.
For ninety minutes, hope had direction.
Attention had an object.
Possibility remained open.
Then the whistle closes all of it.
The equalizer will not come.
The comeback is over.
The future the supporter had been carrying toward the final minutes is suddenly gone.
The loss is not only what happened.
It is also what will not happen now.
And even after the result is fixed, the mind may resist leaving it alone.
One pass.
One miss.

One decision.
What if?
Before kickoff, those words opened possibilities.
After the whistle, they point toward versions of the match that can no longer occur.
The match is fixed.
The alternatives are not.

Later, the match finds its place among everything that surrounded it.

Some experiences fade.

Others remain unexpectedly close.

So do some of the emotions.

So do some of the questions.

The whistle decides the score.
It does not always decide what happens next inside us.

CHAPTER 8 — THE HURT THAT SURPRISES US

The final whistle goes.

For one side, arms rise.

For the other, almost nothing moves.

A player bends forward with his hands on his knees.

Someone sits back down.

A television keeps showing the field, but the room has changed.

A few seconds earlier, there was still somewhere for hope to go.

Now there is not.

The score is final.

That word carries more weight than it seems it should.

The supporter did not take the penalty or concede the goal, yet defeat can still arrive with real force.

The chest feels heavy.

Conversation becomes difficult.

An evening that had been organized around possibility suddenly feels empty.

Sometimes the reaction surprises even the person having it.

How can something that happened on a field, to other people, hurt this much?

The answer begins long before the whistle.

A supporter rarely enters an important match emotionally neutral.

Hours, days, sometimes years have already been invested in what the result could mean.

The team carries identity.

Past matches sit behind the present one.

The competition has a history.

The opponent has a meaning.

The possibility of winning has been imagined before anyone steps onto the field.

By kickoff, the result is no longer just information waiting to arrive.

It is attached to expectation.

That attachment makes losing hurt more.
A neutral observer can watch a final and appreciate the football.
A supporter watches with part of the self-tied to one side of the score.
The same goal can therefore produce two completely different experiences.
For one person, release.
For another, collapse.
Belonging made the result personal long before defeat made the pain visible.
Something emotionally valuable disappears with the loss.
The celebration.
The trophy lift.
The walk home after victory.
Defeat removes all of it at once.
We do not lose only the score.
We can also lose the future we had already begun imagining.
Victory does not need to feel guaranteed.
It only needs to feel possible.
A close final enters the last ten minutes.
The score is level.
One attack could decide it.
Every clearance preserves hope.
Every run forward keeps the imagined celebration alive.
Then a goal arrives at the other end.
The supporter had been carrying one version of the next hour.
Reality replaces it in seconds.
Expectation has momentum.
The mind prepares for what seems likely, possible, or desired.
Emotion leans toward a future before that future exists.
A late defeat can hurt especially sharply because there is so little time to adjust.
At 0–0, many endings remain available.
At 1–0 with twenty minutes left, an equalizer can still be imagined.
At 1–0 with three minutes left, hope narrows but survives.
One chance.
There is still time.
Then the whistle goes.
Nothing remains to negotiate.

A final whistle after defeat does more than stop play.
It removes the last path through which the desired result might still arrive.
The clock had been an ally because time meant possibility.
Now time has run out.
The supporter must move from anticipation to acceptance almost immediately.
A supporter may spend the closing minutes tense, alert, focused on every touch.
Then the whistle sounds.
Attention has nowhere useful to go.
The body had been prepared for another attack.
The mind had been prepared for another chance.
Instead there is closure.
That was it.

The state built for what might happen next cannot simply complete itself. Attention had narrowed. Readiness had risen. The body had been organized around another possibility. When the possibility disappears, that preparation loses its destination before the body has fully let it go.

The drop can feel physical.
Shoulders fall.
Breathing changes.
Noise disappears.
People who had been standing sit down without speaking.
The same room that felt electrically alive minutes earlier can feel strangely flat.
High anticipation organizes the body around what might happen next.
When the desired outcome disappears, that state loses its object.
The result can feel like deflation.
A missed penalty makes the shift especially abrupt.
The player walks toward the ball carrying a possibility.
Score, and the match moves one way.
Miss, and it moves another.
The run-up lasts seconds.
The shot goes wide.
For one side, release is immediate.
For the other, possibility collapses just as quickly.
The mind had already moved toward one ending.

Reality delivers another.

Expectation and outcome collide.

The greater the investment, the harder the correction can feel.

A match watched casually does not produce the same fall as a final waited for all season.

A tournament defeat can land with the weight of weeks of accumulated expectation.

Meaning magnifies consequence.

Brazil's 2014 World Cup semifinal against Germany showed expectation collapsing faster than emotion could adjust.

Brazil entered the match carrying the weight of a home World Cup and the possibility of reaching the final.

Then the game moved away from them with extraordinary speed.

Germany scored repeatedly in the first half.

The expected contest did not merely tilt.

It disappeared.

One goal might have allowed time to adjust.

Then came another.

Then another.

The distance between hope and reality widened almost immediately.

By the time the result was effectively beyond reach, much of the match still remained.

The players kept moving.

The clock kept running.

The television stayed on.

The supporter was still inside the event while already confronting its loss.

Attacks no longer carried the same promise.

Minutes that once seemed scarce could suddenly feel excessive.

The match continued after hope had lost its direction.

Pain is shaped not only by where we end, but by how far the ending sits from the future we had prepared for.

Losing after expecting little can hurt.

Losing after allowing ourselves to picture victory can hurt differently.

Knowing that defeat is possible does not prevent emotional investment in victory.

The hurt reflects how much emotional space the team and the result had come to occupy.

That connection can make disappointment feel personal even when the event itself was not.

A player misses.

A defender hesitates.

A goalkeeper cannot reach the shot.

The supporter may be thousands of miles away.

Still, the loss arrives inwardly.

The language gives it away.

We lost.

The same pronoun that enlarged victory now carries defeat.

The pain shows how fully the outcome had been incorporated into the self.

A neutral spectator closes the match.

A supporter may need time for the emotional state built around it to fall away.

That comedown is often visible in silence.

Not the concentrated silence before a penalty.

A different silence.

Nothing is waiting to happen now.

The question has been answered.

There is no need to hold breath.

No reason to stand.

No next attack capable of changing the result.

The quiet after defeat has a different texture because anticipation has disappeared.

The energy that filled the match has collapsed with it.

Someone turns off the television.

Someone leaves the room.

Someone remains seated for another minute.

The loss can dominate the evening because emotional investment had accumulated long before the score became final.

A season.

A rivalry.

A tournament.

Years of attachment.

The final score concentrates all of it into one answer.

Victory rewards the investment.
Defeat exposes it.
We care.
We anticipate.
We attach ourselves to an outcome.
We begin living slightly ahead of the present.
Then reality arrives.
Sometimes it gives us the future we had imagined.
Sometimes it removes it.
The scoreboard has changed only by a number.
The emotional world around it has changed far more.
The final whistle closes the match.
It also closes the future the supporter had been carrying toward it.
That is what defeat can take.
Not only the game that was played.
The ending that never arrived.

CHAPTER 9 — THE MATCH THAT REFUSES TO END

The match ended twenty minutes ago.

The television is off.

The stadium is emptying.

The score cannot change.

And still, one moment keeps returning.

The pass should have gone left.

The striker should have taken one more touch.

The defender should have stepped forward.

The referee should have seen it.

The ball was inches from the post.

The game is finished.

The alternatives are not.

During a match, imagining what might happen next is useful.

A midfielder receives the ball and several possibilities open.

Pass.

Turn.

Shoot.

Hold possession.

The mind tries to anticipate which one will occur.

Once the action happens, most of those possibilities disappear.

Another set replaces them.

At the final whistle, reality stops producing new football.

The mind does not always stop producing alternatives.

A supporter leaves the match with the result already fixed and begins constructing versions that never occurred.

What if he had passed?

What if the goalkeeper had stayed on his line?

What if the shot had been half a meter lower?

What if the referee had allowed play to continue?

Before the whistle, questions like these point forward.

After it, they point backward.

The same capacity that helps us imagine possible futures can be turned toward a completed past.

The mind takes what happened and places another outcome beside it.

The real pass went right.

The imagined pass goes left.

The real shot struck the post.

The imagined shot enters the goal.

Nothing on the field changes.

The internal match does.

This kind of thinking reaches far beyond football.

A conversation ends and the better response arrives on the way home.

An interview finishes and one answer is mentally rewritten.

Human beings are skilled at generating alternatives to events that have already occurred.

Football gives that habit unusually clear material.

The field is bounded.

The score is known.

The decisive moments are visible.

Many of them turn on tiny differences.

One step.

One touch.

One decision.

A few centimeters.

A shot travels just wide.

The difference between what happened and what might have happened is physically small.

Move the ball slightly.

Change the angle.

Delay the defender by half a second.

The entire emotional result changes.

The closeness of the alternative gives it power.

A shot that misses by ten meters is disappointing.

A shot that clips the outside of the post can haunt the conversation afterward.

The mind can almost see the other outcome.

That word—almost—does a great deal of work.

Almost scored.

Almost saved it.

Almost reached the final.

Almost held on.

A missed penalty offers an especially clean example.

The kick is taken.

The goalkeeper moves.

The ball goes wide.

The result is complete.

But the mind can alter the scene instantly.

A little farther inside the post.

A slightly different run-up.

A calmer finish.

Goal.

The imagined version requires almost no effort because the real event already supplied the structure.

Only one detail needs changing.

That small change can reorganize everything that follows.

The score.

The celebration.

The night.

The mind is drawn toward moments like these because they look editable.

Near misses make alternative endings unusually easy to construct. The mind does not have to invent an entirely different match. Most of reality can remain exactly where it is. Move one pass, one foot, one decision, one piece of the ball—and a different future seems to appear almost intact. The smaller the imagined correction, the more reachable the lost outcome can feel.

A match may contain hundreds of passes, but attention after defeat often returns to the few moments where another outcome seemed nearest.

A referee decision can have the same effect.

The whistle goes.

Play stops.

The replay appears.

From one angle, the contact looks clear.
From another, less so.
The discussion begins before the broadcast has even moved on.
Was it a foul?
Was he offside?
Should advantage have been played?
The official decision is fixed inside the match.
Outside it, interpretation keeps moving.
Different angles supply different evidence.
Memory combines what was seen live with what appears in replay.
Conversation adds other interpretations.
The original moment starts accumulating versions.
A two-second event can occupy an hour of argument.
Someone disagrees.
The replay is shown again.
Another angle changes the interpretation.
The argument begins again.
The match is no longer being played by footballers.
It is being reconstructed in conversation.
Highlights extend that process.

The final whistle has already produced closure, yet the most emotionally charged moments are shown again.

The chance.
The miss.
The save.
The decision.
The goal.

Each replay returns the supporter to a point where, during the match, the outcome had not yet been known.

For a few seconds, the sequence is visible again.
Attention still follows the movement.
The pass arrives.
The striker shoots.
The ball travels toward goal.
The mind knows where it will end.

It can still generate the version in which it ends somewhere else.

Replay reopens the moment for alternatives.

Sometimes that is useful.

The first experience of a decisive moment can be too fast, emotional, or confusing to understand clearly.

Watching again can reveal what was missed.

A defender was covering the runner.

The passing lane was narrower than it looked.

The referee's view was obstructed.

What felt obvious in real time can look different once the sequence is slowed and seen from another angle.

Revisiting the event can turn reaction into understanding.

The supporter updates the story.

He should have passed.

Then the replay shows the defender closing the lane.

Perhaps the shot made sense.

Post-match conversation can do the same.

Another person noticed movement away from the ball.

Someone remembers an earlier tactical change.

The match gains structure after the emotion settles enough to examine it.

But replay can continue after the information stops changing.

The same clip is watched again.

The same argument is repeated.

The same decision is reconstructed.

Nothing new enters.

The alternative remains attractive because it still produces a different ending.

What if he had passed?

The question once invited analysis.

After the tenth repetition, it may simply reopen the loss.

One kind of replay asks:

What happened?

Another asks:

How else could it have ended?

The first can produce understanding.

The second can continue indefinitely.

A football match offers almost unlimited material for that second question.
Change one decision and another sequence appears.
The midfielder passes sooner.
The striker chooses the other corner.
Soon the supporter is no longer reconsidering one moment.
An entire alternative match is being constructed.
This version is seductive because it has no resistance from reality.
The real match had opponents.
Deflections.
Bad touches.
Unexpected decisions.
The imagined one can quietly remove whatever prevented the desired result.
One corrected pass leads to the goal.
One successful penalty changes the night.

The alternative can feel cleaner than the match that actually occurred because it is built backward from the outcome we wanted.
Reality had to unfold forward.
The imagined version already knows where it wants to end.
During the match, prediction works with uncertainty.
No one knows which path will survive.

Afterward, hindsight can make the rejected path look more obvious than it ever was in real time.

The supporter now knows where the danger came from, which pass failed, which decision changed the match.
From the end of the story, another choice can look inevitable.
It rarely felt that inevitable before the outcome arrived.
A midfielder hesitates for half a second and loses the ball.
After the match, the open teammate is easy to see.
Pause the frame.
Point to the space.
There.
Pass there.
But the frozen image contains information the player never possessed in frozen form.
The match was moving.
Opponents were moving.

The decision had to happen before the supporter knew what would follow.

Afterward, knowledge of the result changes the way the earlier moment is judged.

The finished outcome casts a shadow backward.

The score has closure.

Thought does not require it.

The final whistle may have occurred hours earlier.

The body has left the stadium.

Dinner has been eaten.

A conversation has moved to something else.

Then one image returns.

The missed chance.

The open runner.

The shot against the post.

For a moment, the match is present again.

The result is known, yet the mind can still generate another route through it.

There is a point where analysis has given everything it has to give.

The replay has been seen.

The decision has been understood.

The alternative has been named.

No new angle changes it.

No additional conversation reveals anything different.

The match is still being replayed, but it is no longer being learned from.

At that point, continuing does not make the past more understandable.

It only keeps the past active.

The game has already taken ninety minutes.

It does not need the rest of the night.

The score is fixed.

The missed chance is fixed.

The decision is fixed.

Understanding may require looking back.

Living forward eventually requires leaving the result where it happened.

The mind can imagine an endless number of matches that were never played.

Only one reached the final whistle.

CHAPTER 10 — THE PLACE WE RETURN TO

You walk into a room you have not seen for years.
The furniture has changed.
The television is different.
Someone has repainted the walls.
And still, something feels familiar before you can say why.
Then it returns.
A match.
A goal.
A voice from the other side of the room.
Someone standing where the table used to be.
For a moment, the place is carrying more than what is physically there.
Football memories often behave like this.
We remember the event.
We also remember where life placed us when it happened.
A particular sofa.
A crowded café.
A family home.
A shirt worn that evening.
A song heard before kickoff.
One of those things can bring the match close again long after the final whistle.
Memory does not attach itself only to events.
It attaches itself to where and how those events were lived.
A football match arrives surrounded by context.
The screen has a position in the room.
Certain people are nearby.
There is light outside the window.
Someone is sitting in the usual chair.

These details are present while the experience unfolds, and some remain tied to it.

The mind does not store every experience as an isolated event floating free of its surroundings.

People, places, sounds, objects, and routines can become part of the context through which an experience is remembered.

A match therefore acquires more than a score.

It acquires a setting.

Think of a final watched at home.

The football itself may happen thousands of miles away.

Long afterward, the remembered night may begin with the room.

The position of the television.

The person sitting beside you.

The place where someone stood during a penalty.

The doorway through which another person entered just before the goal.

The stadium may have held the players.

The living room held your experience of them.

A stadium is an obvious football place.

It has stands, floodlights, gates, songs, seats, and a pitch.

Its purpose is visible.

But a room can become a football place without looking like one.

So can a café.

A kitchen.

A neighborhood street.

A family home.

Nothing about the architecture needs to announce what happened there.

The memory supplies that part.

A café may be ordinary on Monday morning.

Tables.

Cups.

People passing through.

Then someone who watched a decisive match there returns.

The room carries another version beneath the present one.

That was where we were.

That corner was crowded.

Someone dropped a glass when the goal went in.

People who had never met were shouting together.

The café has returned to normal.

Memory has not made it ordinary again.

Places acquire emotional history through repetition as well as singular events.

A supporter may watch dozens of matches from the same chair.

At first, it is simply where the television can be seen clearly.

Over time, different nights accumulate there.

Wins.

Defeats.

A comeback.

A final.

The chair remains physically unchanged while its associations multiply.

Eventually, sitting there before kickoff can carry traces of earlier matches without any deliberate attempt to remember them.

The present location activates part of its own history.

A street can remind someone of childhood before a specific memory appears.

A song can return a person to a particular summer.

The smell of a familiar house can make years feel unexpectedly close.

Context gives memory routes back into experience.

Recall does not always begin with a deliberate search. Sometimes a cue activates part of an old experience before the rest has returned. One detail reaches another. The room brings back a voice. The voice brings back the match. The match brings back the person you were when you watched it. Memory can rebuild a larger world from a surprisingly small entrance.

Football repeatedly uses the same routes because matches return.

The same rooms.

The same routes home.

The same cafés.

The same people.

Repetition creates layers.

Then one extraordinary match can dominate them.

A supporter may watch fifty matches in one room and remember one night far more vividly than the others.

The room becomes linked to that night because emotion gave certain details unusual staying power.

The cue does not need to be dramatic.

A lamp in the corner.

A particular view from the window.

The sound of dishes from another room.

One detail can open a larger scene.

Objects can work the same way.

A football shirt begins as fabric.

Then it is worn during matches.

Photographs are taken in it.

Someone celebrates in it.

Someone travels in it.

A season passes.

Much later, the shirt may be folded in a drawer long after the players once associated with it have left the club.

Take it out and the object carries more than its design.

It may carry a period of life.

The apartment where matches were watched.

The friends who used to come over.

The person who gave the shirt as a gift.

The object has remained while the life around it has moved on.

A scarf can do the same.

So can a ticket.

A photograph.

The match disappears as soon as it is played.

The object stays.

Its continued presence gives memory something physical to attach to.

Songs work differently.

They can disappear completely and then return without warning.

A few notes begin.

Recognition is immediate.

Before the lyrics are fully conscious, another place may already be coming back.

A road toward a match.

A crowded room.

A tournament summer.

Music can carry entire periods of life because it often repeats around the same experiences.

A song heard throughout one tournament can become difficult to separate from the tournament itself.

Hear it again and it may bring back more than football.

Age.

Friends.

A city.

The person you were at the time.

Football memory easily crosses into autobiographical memory because football happens inside ordinary life.

People watch while growing up.

While studying.

While working.

While moving between cities.

While friendships change.

While people leave.

A club may remain on the screen while almost everything around the screen changes.

That continuity gives football an unusual ability to mark time.

One shirt belongs to school years.

Another to a first apartment.

One tournament belongs to a particular summer.

The score is part of the memory.

So is the life surrounding it.

Years can therefore be organized by matches without anyone deliberately using football as a calendar.

Mention a season and another memory appears beside it.

That was when we lived there.

That was before they moved away.

That was the summer we watched every match together.

That was the year the café on the corner was still open.

The football provides a date.

Life supplies the meaning around it.

Neighborhoods can gather this kind of memory collectively.

A street after an important victory looks like the same street.

The buildings have not moved.
The pavement is unchanged.
But windows open.
Cars sound their horns.
Children stay awake later than usual.
For a few hours, an ordinary route acquires another identity.

Return to the same street much later and the noise can come back before anything visible has changed.
The memory supplies the crowd.
One supporter remembers where he stood.
Another remembers who called.
Someone else remembers leaning from a window.

The street belongs to everyone, but each person carries a slightly different version of that night.
Family homes hold especially dense versions of these memories.
Football may enter through repetition rather than spectacle.
Weekend matches in the same room.
A parent commenting from the same chair.
Children learning when the adults become quiet.
Meals delayed because the second half has started.
The details seem ordinary while they are happening.
Their ordinariness can later become part of their emotional force.
The match is remembered because the people are remembered with it.
A scoreline can survive beside a voice that is no longer heard every day.
A competition can bring back the arrangement of a room that no longer exists.
Football forms one thread through a larger autobiographical memory.
It does not simply return us to an event.
It returns us toward a former version of life.

The old shirt, café, or television mattered because they were present while a particular life was being lived.
Memory gathered around them.
Return later, and the football may be the first thing that surfaces.
Underneath it is something larger.
Who was there.
How old you were.

What the weekends felt like.

What had not changed yet.

A familiar match-day route can produce the same effect.

It may lead from home to a friend's house.

Or from an apartment to a café.

Walked often enough, it acquires sequence.

This corner means almost there.

This street was always busy before kickoff.

The route gathers expectation before matches and memories after them.

Walk it again after enough time has passed, and an old match day can feel unexpectedly close.

The memory may arrive before the specific game does.

First comes familiarity.

Then atmosphere.

Then perhaps one night separates itself from the others.

A result.

A celebration.

Someone who was there.

Context can work in both directions.

A place can call back a match.

A match can call back a place.

Mention a famous goal and someone remembers a room.

Mention a tournament and someone sees a summer street.

Hear an old song and suddenly the café is full again.

Football history is never only the history recorded in stadiums.

For supporters, much of it happened elsewhere.

On sofas.

Around tables.

In cafés.

In bedrooms long after everyone else had gone to sleep.

In streets where celebration arrived through open windows.

The official record contains the score, the scorer, the minute, the competition.

Personal memory keeps different statistics.

Who was there.

Where you stood.

Which room erupted.

Which voice you can still hear.

Two people can remember the same goal and carry entirely different places inside it.

One was in the stadium.

One was at home with family.

One was alone in another country.

The event is shared.

The remembered world around it is personal.

Returning to a place can sometimes feel like returning to football even when no match is being played.

The screen is dark.

The café is quiet.

The street is empty.

The old shirt is hanging in a closet.

Nothing is happening now.

And still, the place can feel occupied by another time.

Memory has given geography an emotional dimension.

A room can hold a final.

A street can hold a celebration.

A shirt can hold a season.

A song can hold a summer.

Football turns ordinary surroundings into landmarks without changing their physical shape.

The match ends.

The room remains.

Years later, we may return to the room.

And find the match still there.

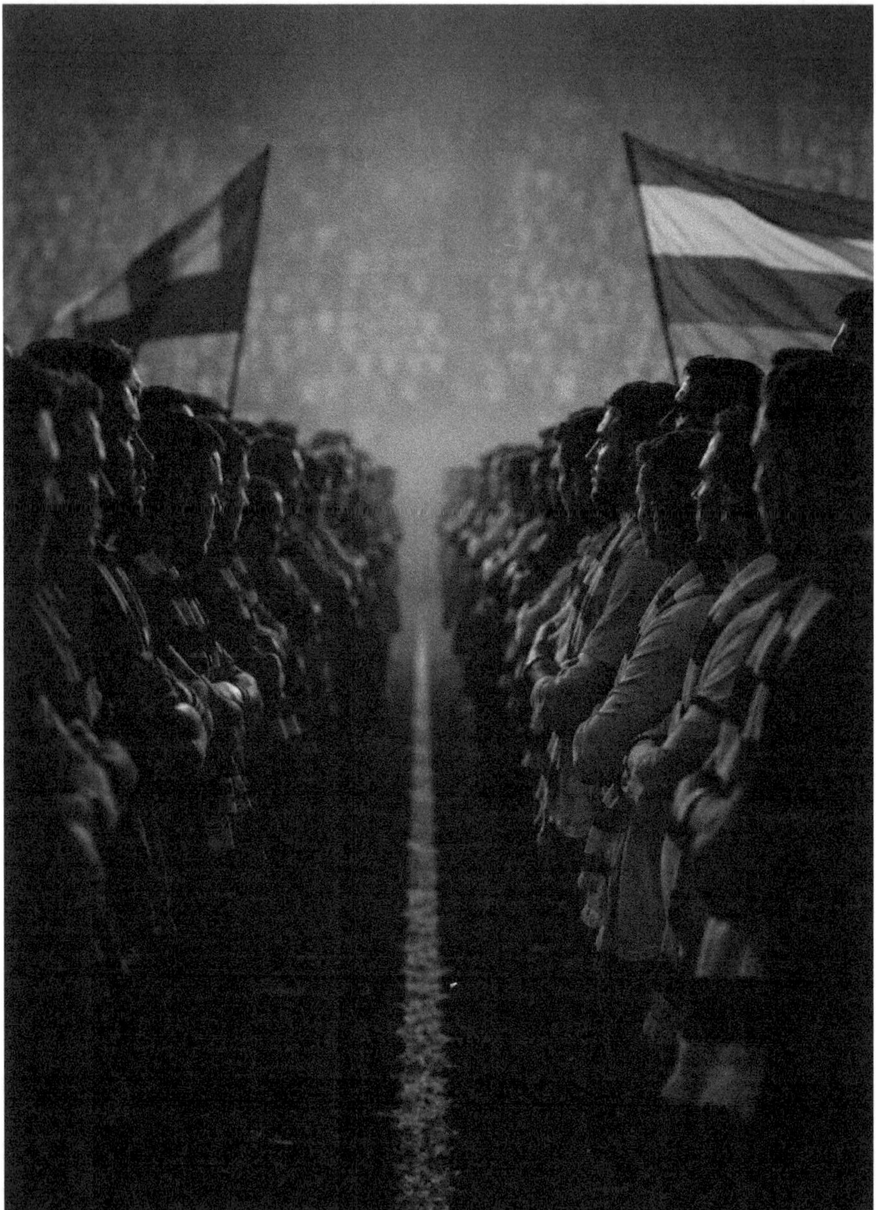

PART IV — BEYOND THE GAME

What Belonging, Attachment, Loss, and Hope Reveal About Us

By now, football has done more than entertain.

It has entered attention.

Changed the body.

Distorted time.

Joined strangers.

Hurt after the whistle.

Stayed in the mind.

Attached itself to places and years.

The match may take place inside white lines, but almost everything that gives it emotional force reaches beyond them.

Belonging is part of that force.

So is attachment.

To care about a team is to allow events elsewhere to acquire personal weight.

A result can enter the evening.

A memory can survive for decades.

A word as small as *we* can pull strangers closer.

But *we* never exists alone.

The moment there is an inside, there is also an outside.

Belonging can pull people together.

The same boundary can also push people apart.

One side wants what the other side cannot have.

The same moment can carry joy in one direction and disappointment in another.

Attachment gives the game its depth.

It also gives the game leverage over us.

The deeper the attachment, the more football can give.

The deeper the attachment, the more it can take.

Still, people return.

The old result remains fixed.

The future does not.

Human beings live by attaching themselves to things that cannot be fully controlled.

People.

Groups.

Ambitions.

Outcomes.

Futures.

We invest without guarantees.

We hope.

We carry disappointment.

We continue.

Football matters.

The harder question is how much space any one result should be allowed to occupy.

The game asks us to care.

Life eventually asks us to know where that caring belongs.

We belong.

We divide.

We lose.

We remember.

We return.

And somehow, despite knowing what the game can do to us, we still return.

CHAPTER 11 — THE OTHER SIDE OF "WE"

The foul happens near the touchline.
Two players arrive at the ball almost together.
One goes down.
The referee blows the whistle.
Half the stadium rises in anger.
The other half applauds the decision.
They have watched the same contact.
Seen the same bodies collide.
Heard the same whistle.
And somehow they have not seen the same event.
One side sees a clear foul.
The other sees a player throwing himself to the ground.
One sees protection from the referee.
The other sees injustice.
The replay appears.
The argument survives it.
Slow motion does not always produce agreement.
Sometimes it gives disagreement more material.
Football is full of moments like this.
A tackle.
A handball.
An offside line.
A penalty appeal.
The event itself may last only seconds.
What follows can divide thousands of people almost instantly.
The division begins with a small word.

We.

In football, *we* can create warmth with remarkable speed.
A stranger wearing the same shirt may receive a smile before a word is spoken.
A goal can send people who have never met into one another's arms.

A shared badge can make an unfamiliar face feel familiar.

But every *we* creates a boundary.

There is someone on the other side of it.

They.

Once that boundary carries emotion, perception does not always remain neutral.

A supporter watches an opponent arrive late in a tackle.

Reckless.

Dangerous.

Unnecessary.

Ten minutes later, one of his own players arrives with similar force.

Committed.

Strong.

He got the ball.

The difference may be smaller on the field than it feels in the stands.

Identity has entered the judgment.

Groups carry histories.

Symbols.

Stories.

Memories.

Famous victories.

Humiliating defeats.

A rival club is never only eleven players in different shirts.

It may carry decades of accumulated meaning before the match begins.

A fixture between unfamiliar teams can start at zero.

A rivalry rarely does.

The past enters with the players.

Old matches sit behind the new one.

A controversial decision from years earlier may still be remembered.

A famous goal may still be celebrated.

A defeat may still irritate people who were children when it happened.

Each new meeting arrives inside an existing story.

The opponent is already known.

Or believed to be.

They are arrogant.

They play dirty.

They get every decision.

Supporters on the other side often possess a parallel story.

About us.

Group identity can turn millions of individuals into categories.

The people wearing one color feel more similar to one another.

Those wearing another are easier to describe as a single thing.

A stadium may contain thousands of different personalities, families, histories, temperaments, and beliefs.

For ninety minutes, much of that complexity can be compressed into two pronouns.

Us.

Them.

That compression makes belonging possible at scale.

No supporter needs to know everyone in the stand before feeling connected to them.

The badge does part of the work.

The colors do part of the work.

The shared outcome does the rest.

But compression removes detail.

The other side is easier to judge collectively.

One supporter behaves badly.

Soon the story shifts:

They are like that.

One player exaggerates contact.

They always cheat.

Individual behavior spreads across the category.

The same generosity is rarely applied inward.

Bad behavior on our side is treated as an exception.

He does not represent us.

Bad behavior on the other side can become evidence.

He reveals them.

Football makes this asymmetry unusually visible because the categories are marked so clearly.

Colors.

Badges.

Songs.

Flags.

The boundary can be seen from across the pitch.

National football can rearrange it.

A tournament begins and people divided by club loyalties suddenly stand beneath the same flag.

Rivals become teammates.

Supporters who argued all season now want the same result.

The scale of *we* has expanded.

That larger identity can produce extraordinary solidarity.

Cities fill with flags.

Families organize their days around matches.

People who rarely speak to one another find immediate common ground.

For a few weeks, a national team can provide millions of people with one emotional calendar.

But enlargement does not remove the boundary.

It moves it.

The club rival who was *them* last month may now be part of *us*.

Another nation takes the opposite position.

A supporter may dislike a player fiercely during the club season and defend the same player passionately when he wears the national shirt.

The person has not changed.

The category has.

So has the emotional interpretation.

Hostility does not live permanently inside the other person.

It depends partly on the relationship between identities.

The same player can move from outsider to insider with a transfer.

The same supporters can move from opponents to allies when the national team plays.

The same behavior can acquire a different meaning once the shirt changes.

A hard tackle from a rival can look cynical.

From a player wearing our colors, it can look brave.

A celebration from the other side can feel provocative.

The same intensity from our side can look like passion.

The behavior is filtered through allegiance before judgment finishes forming.

Perception and interpretation do not arrive as perfectly separate stages. The mind is already assigning meaning while the event is still being understood. Identity supplies part of that context. Once an action carries consequences for us, the same evidence can feel different before we have consciously decided why.

Referees stand directly inside this problem.

They are expected to occupy a position no supporter can fully occupy during an emotionally important match.

Neutrality.

The referee sees contact.

Supporters see contact plus consequence.

If the whistle harms the team we care about, the decision arrives carrying emotional cost.

That cost can influence how the decision is interpreted.

A marginal foul against a neutral team may disappear from memory within minutes.

The same foul against our team in a decisive match can survive for years.

The replay is watched again.

Angles are compared.

Frames are paused.

Certainty may increase inside each group.

Our side was robbed.

Their side got away with it.

More replay does not guarantee convergence when identity shapes what the evidence means.

One angle shows contact.

Was it enough?

Another shows the player beginning to fall.

Did he exaggerate?

The evidence expands.

So does interpretation.

The supporter often wants the answer that preserves the story already being carried.

We were treated unfairly.

They benefited.

We deserved more.

A disputed penalty begins with contact between two players.
Minutes later, the conversation may contain claims about an entire club.
Their players are always like this.
Their club has always been favored.
One incident expands to fill a much older story.
Rivalries give incidents somewhere ready to land.
The event enters a structure already waiting for it.
Online spaces accelerate the process.
Inside a stadium, an argument has physical limits.
The match ends.
People leave.
Distance increases.
Online, the incident can keep circulating.
A ten-second clip appears without the minutes surrounding it.
A still image freezes the most incriminating frame.
A caption supplies an interpretation before the viewer presses play.
Disagreement arrives underneath.
So does ridicule.
So does certainty.
Groups gather around versions of the event that already match what they believe.
The loudest interpretation travels.
Sarcasm sharpens it.
Anger rewards anger.

A supporter who begins mildly irritated can spend twenty minutes reading hundreds of people confirming that the decision was disgraceful.

Emotion gains company.
The individual reaction starts feeling like consensus.
The other side is doing the same thing elsewhere.
Two groups can move farther apart after the match is over.
Each side encounters evidence filtered through people who share its allegiance.
Each sees the other side at its least charitable.
A foolish post from one rival supporter is captured and circulated.
Look at them.
A hostile comment receives thousands of responses.

This is what they are like.
The category grows simpler as the emotional temperature rises.
A crowd contains people of every temperament and history.
Rivalry can flatten that complexity.
The rival badge arrives first.
Everything else moves behind it.
Chants make the boundary audible.
Many begin playfully.
Mockery is part of rivalry.
One stand sings.
The other answers.
Humor travels across the stadium.
The exchange gives the match another layer.
But group emotion can escalate.
One chant hardens.
The response hardens with it.
Someone finds the next insult.

Thousands repeat words many of them would never say alone to a stranger in an ordinary setting.

The group changes what feels permissible.
A person who would hesitate privately may join publicly.
Responsibility feels more distributed.
The chant is already moving.
Others are singing.
The individual voice disappears inside the collective one.
Shared emotion does not amplify only joy.
Anger can gather voices too.
Contempt can find rhythm.
Hostility is easier when it arrives surrounded by agreement.
The social environment changes the threshold for joining.
One voice creates little pressure.
A thousand voices make participation feel normal.
The boundary between teams now has sound.
Sometimes the escalation remains ritualized.
The match ends.

The chant ends.
Supporters leave.
At other times, the emotion travels farther.
A thrown object.
A confrontation outside the ground.
Abuse directed at a player.
The distance between rivalry and hostility can be crossed through accumulation.
A perceived injustice.
An insult.
Another provocation.
Each moment changes the emotional context for the next one.
What might have been ignored earlier now feels like evidence of disrespect.
The other group's reaction confirms the negative story already forming.
They hate us.
They are arrogant.
They deserve whatever comes back.
Once actions are interpreted through that frame, escalation can feed itself.
A gesture becomes a provocation.
A celebration becomes an insult.
Silence becomes disrespect.
Ambiguous behavior is pulled toward the interpretation the group is already prepared to see.
People do not need to consciously decide to distort reality.
They care about the outcome.
They care about the identity.
They want one story to be true more than another.
That preference can influence which evidence feels convincing.
Imagine the same close handball appeal shown to two groups of supporters.
The ball strikes an arm.
The arm is away from the body, but not dramatically.
One group immediately sees a penalty.
The other sees unavoidable contact.
Both can produce reasons.
Distance.

Movement.

Position.

Precedent.

The arguments sound objective.

Emotion may already have selected the preferred destination.

Neutral matches can feel mentally quieter.

A supporter may still disagree with a decision.

But less identity is at stake.

The interpretation can remain flexible.

Perhaps it was a foul.

Perhaps not.

When the decision threatens *us*, uncertainty can feel harder to tolerate.

Certainty protects the group.

We were right.

We were wronged.

They benefited.

The story remains intact.

Group identity can also shape memory.

Supporters remember famous injustices committed against their side.

Incidents that benefited them often acquire less historical weight.

A rivalry can therefore develop two archives.

Each side carries a collection of evidence proving the other has been favored, dishonest, arrogant, or protected.

The archives rarely contain the same moments.

Each generation inherits parts of them.

Stories are retold.

Children learn which defeats still hurt.

Which players are still disliked.

Which decisions still provoke anger.

A person can enter a rivalry long after the original event and receive its emotional meaning almost immediately.

The memory is carried socially.

We remember what happened to us.

They remember what happened to them.

The two histories can occupy the same years and barely resemble one another.

Moral double standards grow easily inside these competing histories.
When our player wastes time near the corner flag, he is intelligent.
When theirs does it, he is disgraceful.
Our striker knows how to win contact.
Theirs dives.
The vocabulary changes before the behavior does.
Humor often exposes the contradiction because supporters recognize it in themselves.

A fan can condemn time-wasting for eighty-five minutes and celebrate it enthusiastically in the final five once his team leads.
The principle did not change.
The desired outcome did.
Football makes a common human tendency unusually visible.
People protect identities they value.
They interpret threats differently when those threats are directed inward.
They forgive insiders more readily.
They generalize from outsiders more quickly.
The shirt makes the process visible.

Take the shirt away and similar tendencies can appear around nations, professions, beliefs, or families.
Football gives the boundary a scoreboard.
The result gives opposing groups a direct relationship.
For us to advance, they may need to go home.
For us to lift the trophy, they must lose the final.
For our goal to produce joy, someone else must experience disappointment.
Competition places conflicting desires inside the same event.
The problem begins when the opposition required by the game expands beyond the game.
A rival supporter becomes a category rather than an individual.
A disputed call becomes evidence of conspiracy.
A loss becomes permission for abuse.
At that point, the boundary has traveled farther than the ball ever needed it to.
The boundary itself is part of football's emotional structure.
The badge matters because another badge stands opposite it.
Victory has shape because defeat exists beside it.
Opposition creates stakes.

But the same boundary that organizes competition can also organize judgment.

A shared identity can widen generosity inward.

It can narrow generosity outward.

The same boundary produces both.

The word *we* still carries warmth.

It still carries memory.

It still allows a person sitting thousands of miles away to feel connected to people never met.

But *we* casts a shadow.

There is always someone outside the pronoun.

Football makes that shadow visible every time two teams walk onto the same field.

Two sets of colors.

Two songs.

Two histories.

Two desired endings.

One ball.

The match asks them to oppose one another.

The rivalry can remain fierce without requiring the person on the other side to disappear inside the category.

Every *we* creates a boundary.

Football shows how powerful that boundary can be.

It also shows how easily we can forget that the people on the other side are saying *we* too.

CHAPTER 12 — WHY WE ALWAYS COME BACK

The defeat felt final on Sunday.

By Wednesday, someone is checking the next fixture.

Not with great enthusiasm.

Not yet.

The result still irritates.

The missed chance still appears in conversation.

Perhaps the referee decision has been watched one more time.

Nothing about the previous match has changed.

And still, the next one has started to acquire shape.

Saturday.

Three o'clock.

Home.

A different opponent.

Someone says:

Maybe we can win that one.

There it is.

Hope has returned before anyone invited it back.

Football produces this strange recovery again and again.

A supporter can leave a stadium insisting that the season is finished, the team is hopeless, the manager has lost control, and there is no reason to expect anything different.

Then a few days pass.

A player returns from injury.

Someone mentions that the next opponent has been struggling.

The predicted lineup looks slightly better.

One small piece of information opens a door that had seemed closed.

Perhaps.

That word has carried football supporters through a remarkable amount of disappointment.

Perhaps the striker finally scores.
Perhaps the defense holds.
Perhaps the opponent has a bad day.
Perhaps this match is different.
A finished match has one ending.
A future match has many.
Hope lives in that gap.
It does not require certainty.
Certainty would almost make hope unnecessary.
Hope requires possibility.
A supporter may know perfectly well that the team is inconsistent.
The evidence may be poor.
Three defeats in four matches.
An injured defender.
A difficult away fixture.
Still, the mind can construct a path.
Keep the first twenty minutes quiet.
Maybe the striker only needs one chance.
Victory does not need to feel likely.
Only available.
Football supplies that possibility with extraordinary regularity.
The calendar keeps producing another date.
One match closes.
Another appears.
Expectation has somewhere to point again.
Memory and hope can coexist.
The supporter may remember the loss perfectly.
A painful defeat can remain painful while another match slowly becomes interesting.
The mind can carry both:
We were terrible last week.
And:
We might win on Saturday.
One statement belongs to the past.
The other belongs to a future that has not yet answered.

The past remains fixed.

The future reopens.

A new season makes the reset more visible.

The final match of the previous year ends.

The table is complete.

The trophy has gone somewhere.

Promotion and relegation have been decided.

For a while, there is nothing left to change.

Then summer rearranges the emotional landscape.

A player signs.

A young player impresses in preseason.

Fixtures are announced.

Training photographs appear.

The old season remains exactly where it ended.

Attention starts drifting forward.

The supporter who spent May saying that nothing would improve finds himself studying August.

Who do we play first?

When is the first home match?

Will the new signing start?

The evidence is still thin.

Imagination has room again.

A new year begins with fewer facts than the old one ended with.

The team that finished tenth can imagine sixth.

The side that barely survived can imagine stability.

The club that lost a final can imagine returning.

The supporter is entering an unwritten space.

Hope often grows there.

A new player can carry an unreasonable amount of that space.

One signing arrives.

Perhaps the supporter has seen highlights.

A few goals.

A few passes.

The first training session has barely ended.

Already futures assemble around him.

He could solve the midfield.

He could change the way the team plays.

He may do neither.

Supporters know how often new signings fail to match the futures imagined for them.

They still imagine.

The new player offers something the old evidence cannot yet cancel.

He has not failed here.

Not yet.

Possibility arrives before performance.

Maybe this is the one.

Sometimes even less is required.

A young player receives a few late minutes, beats a defender, and plays one unexpected pass.

The crowd notices.

The sample is tiny.

The future is large.

Human beings can build expectation from remarkably little when the desired outcome remains possible.

Football keeps supplying fresh material.

A player.

A formation.

A return from injury.

A run of fixtures.

One reason can be enough to reopen the argument with despair.

Football also rewards inconsistently.

Imagine a team that always won.

Not usually.

Always.

Every match.

Every competition.

Every year.

The supporter could still admire the football.

History could still matter.

But victory would stop arriving as surprise.

Relief would weaken.

Possibility would narrow into expectation.

The emotional swing between frustration and reward would flatten.

Football rarely offers that certainty.

Even dominant teams lose.

Weak teams sometimes beat strong ones.

A player out of form suddenly scores twice.

A team that has looked lifeless for weeks produces one magnificent afternoon.

Reward does not arrive on a reliable schedule.

That irregularity gives it force.

The mind pays close attention to rewards that remain possible but cannot be perfectly predicted. Certainty requires little monitoring. Uncertainty keeps the next outcome alive. When reward finally arrives after frustration, its value is shaped not only by the reward itself but by everything that preceded it.

The supporter cannot know which match will provide the moment worth remembering.

Perhaps it is the next one.

A season contains long stretches that disappear quickly.

Then one afternoon produces something else.

A late winner.

A comeback.

A victory nobody expected.

The reward does more than improve the table.

It refreshes belief.

A supporter who had been emotionally withdrawing remembers what the attachment can feel like when it gives something back.

The next match looks different.

The sequence is interrupted.

Pain is interrupted by reward.

Frustration is interrupted by beauty.

Predictability is interrupted by surprise.

The team disappoints again.

Then gives something nobody expected.

Attachment survives inside that uneven pattern.

A supporter may complain precisely because the relationship still matters.

Indifference sounds different.

Indifference does not spend Monday discussing the missed chance.

It does not check the transfer news.

It does not wonder whether Saturday might be different.

Frustration often contains continued investment.

The supporter wants the team to stop disappointing because some part of him still expects the relationship to give something worth returning for.

That expectation can weaken.

It can disappear for a while.

People stop watching every match.

They turn off notifications.

They lose interest during a terrible season.

Some attachments fade completely.

Others move in and out of intensity.

A supporter who stops watching in March may care again in August.

Someone who leaves a final devastated may find himself discussing tactics days later.

The emotion does not always need to be summoned.

The fixture does some of the work.

A familiar badge appears.

A lineup is announced.

The broadcast begins.

The players walk out.

A new match presents itself.

The old story remains behind it.

The new one has not been written.

Maybe this time.

At kickoff, football performs one of its simplest acts of renewal.

The score is 0–0.

Whatever happened last week, this match begins without a goal already conceded.

Whatever was missed in the final belongs to another night.

Whatever anger followed the previous whistle, the next ninety minutes have not yet chosen their meaning.

A fresh kickoff does not erase history.

It temporarily restores openness.

The supporter can once again ask:

What happens next?
The question has appeared before a dangerous pass.
Before a penalty.
Before a final.
Now it carries something larger.
What happens next after everything that has already happened?
Football keeps offering the same answer:
There is another match.
Human beings do not live only through completed events.
We orient toward what is still possible.
Football is structured around recurrence.
Another fixture is built into the competition.
Another season follows this one.
Another tournament waits beyond the current cycle.
The supporter does not have to invent the next opportunity.
The calendar supplies it.
But people do not return only because victory remains possible.
Football gives rewards beyond winning.
The familiar voices.
The shared messages before kickoff.
The walk toward wherever the match will be watched.
The moment when a room rises together.
The possibility that something ordinary may suddenly become memorable.
Attachment contains routine, belonging, recognition, and continuity.
It gives people reasons to call one another.
Dates around which friends gather.
A familiar club that remains present while jobs, cities, homes, and relationships change.
A season may fail competitively and still acquire personal meaning.
A simple calculation of pleasure and pain cannot fully describe loyalty.
Football asks for investment without guaranteeing success in return.

Yet the attachment has been producing value all along—in belonging, memory, continuity, and shared experience.

The club matters even when it loses.
And the next match might still be won.

Memory helps hope in another way.
A supporter approaching a difficult match does not carry only defeats.
The archive contains exceptions.
The comeback nobody expected.
The season that changed after a terrible start.
The victory that seemed impossible at halftime.
Those memories are evidence too.
Not evidence that the next miracle will happen.
Evidence that football has violated expectations before.
A stronger opponent should win.
Usually.
A two-goal deficit should be enough.
Often.
A bad run should continue.
Perhaps.
But memory can supply one stubborn counterexample.
We have seen stranger things.
That sentence gives hope somewhere to stand.
The supporter does not need to believe history will repeat.
Only to remember that certainty has failed before.
The game has trained supporters not to trust closure too early.
A team can look finished and score.
A tournament can look lost and turn.
A player can look hopeless and recover form.
The future remains capable of embarrassing the forecast.
Hope regenerates from two directions.
Time softens the emotional force of one disappointment.
Memory preserves evidence that another outcome is possible.
Then the next fixture arrives.
The supporter returns because the game keeps producing unfinished space ahead.
The next match starts at zero.
The same team may disappoint again.
The new signing may fail.
The promising season may collapse.

The comeback may never arrive.

Hope is not a promise.

It is permission to imagine another outcome.

Football grants that permission repeatedly.

A date appears.

The week begins leaning toward it.

Someone checks the team news.

A conversation starts.

The lineup arrives.

The players walk out.

A ball rests at the center spot.

For a few seconds, the entire history of disappointment exists behind the supporter.

In front of him, nothing has happened yet.

The referee checks the watch.

The whistle sounds.

The ball moves.

And once again, the future is open.

The Emotional Contract

Hope has another side.

We care deeply about things we cannot control.

Football makes that especially clear.

A supporter invests in an outcome without possessing it.

The team may win.

It may lose.

A striker may score.

The chance may disappear.

A decision may go the other way.

For ninety minutes, all of it can feel enormous.

It should.

A final watched from emotional distance would lose something.

A late winner would mean less if part of us remained detached in case disappointment followed.

The embrace after a goal would be smaller if nobody had allowed himself to need the goal in the first place.

Football asks for investment before it reveals the outcome.

That is the bargain.

Belonging comes with vulnerability.

Hope comes with uncertainty.

Shared joy exists because there was something to lose.

The deeper the attachment, the greater the range of what the game can give us.

The same depth enlarges what it can take.

The answer is not less feeling.

The feeling needs somewhere to end.

A match on Saturday can begin consuming Thursday.

Then Wednesday.

Anticipation is part of the pleasure.

The coming fixture creates something to imagine, discuss, and wait for.

But anticipation can make Saturday feel different without taking possession of Friday.

The match has not happened yet.

The rest of life has.

Victory creates a different temptation.

There are moments when football should fill the room.

The final minute of a final.

A penalty shootout.

A goal waited for across years.

Celebrate it.

Shout.

Stand up.

Call someone.

Remember it.

The team won.

That can be enough.

Victory does not need to prove anything larger.

Its value can remain inside the joy of what happened.

Defeat asks something harder.

Let it hurt.

The silence after the whistle is real.

So is the disappointment.

A future that had been imagined has disappeared.

Perhaps the season has ended.

Perhaps the chance will not return for years.

Pain can be real without being permanent.

The match can take the evening.

It does not automatically deserve the next morning.

Sometimes it follows us anyway.

A missed chance returns while driving.

A decision reappears at dinner.

The mind goes back.

What if?

Replay can continue while it teaches something.

A second look may change the interpretation.

A conversation may reveal what emotion concealed in real time.

But when nothing new arrives, the match has already given everything it can give.

The same replay cannot change the result.

The same argument cannot reopen the field.

At some point, looking back stops producing understanding and starts extending the loss.

The game has already taken ninety minutes.

It does not need the rest of the night.

Rivalry has its own boundary.

Football needs opposition.

One side wants what the other side wants.

Only one can have it.

That tension gives the contest much of its force.

The badge can matter.

The disagreement can remain fierce.

The game needs an opponent.

It does not need an enemy in every part of life.

The game can matter deeply without becoming the measure of your life.

Care enough for the result to matter.

Keep enough proportion for the result to remain a result.

Football can enter memory without controlling identity.

It can shape a weekend without defining a person.

It can create joy without needing victory to become evidence of personal worth.

Its scale should remain honest.

A match is powerful partly because its boundaries are so clear.

White lines.

A whistle.

A clock.

Kickoff.

Full time.

Inside them, an attack can feel urgent.

A goal can feel enormous.

One result can briefly seem like the only result that matters.

Then the whistle goes.

The field remains.

The rest of life is still there.

Some things deserve to travel beyond the final whistle.

The joy.
The memory.
The belonging.
The beauty.
The hope.
A goal should survive.
A friendship should survive.
A night of extraordinary football may remain vivid decades later.
Other things may need a shorter journey.
The anger.
The tenth replay of the missed penalty.
The referee decision already examined from every angle.
Those can remain where the match left them.
Understanding may take time.
Eventually, attention has somewhere else to go.
There is another person in the room.
Another conversation.
Another morning.
Another responsibility.
A life that existed before kickoff and continued while the match was being played.
Football can return to its place without losing its meaning.
Not between supporter and team.
Not between *us* and *them*.
Between the game and everything around it.
Know where the game ends and the rest of life resumes.
Then care.
Care enough to feel the body tighten before the chance.
Care enough to stand when the shot leaves the foot.
Care enough to celebrate with strangers.
Care enough for defeat to hurt.
Care enough to remember.

And when the whistle has gone, the result is fixed, and nothing more can be learned from returning to the same moment, allow the rest of life to become visible again.

The game does not need to own everything in order to mean something.
It only needs the space in which we choose to care.

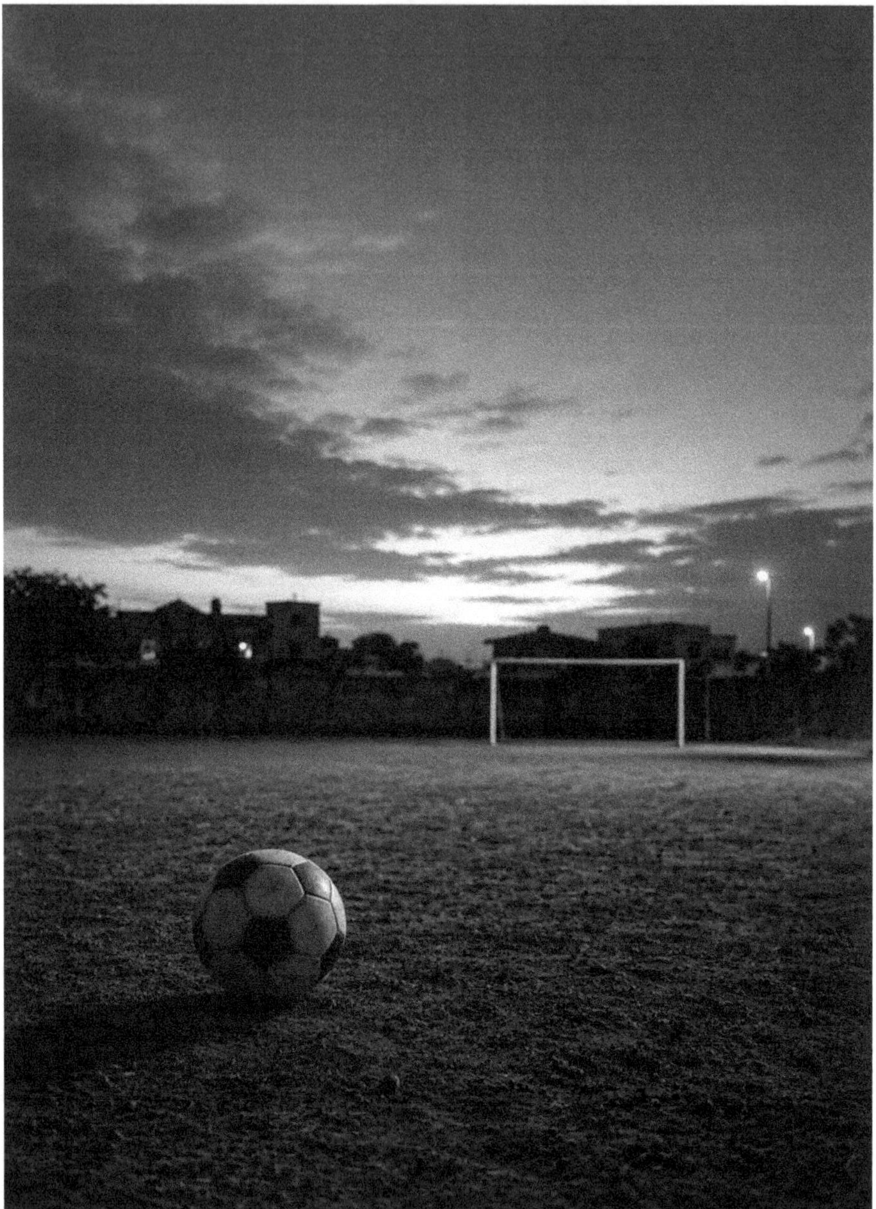

EPILOGUE — THE NEXT KICKOFF

Somewhere, a ball is waiting.

On a patch of grass between two improvised goals.

At the center of a stadium filling with noise.

On a television screen in a room where someone has arrived early.

Outside a café where chairs have been turned toward the match.

The game keeps beginning in different places.

A child watches without knowing everything yet.

The rules are still arriving.

The names are still new.

Perhaps the child notices the people first.

Someone leans forward.

Someone becomes quiet.

A voice rises.

The child looks up.

Nearby, an adult has seen hundreds of matches.

Enough to remember goals that once seemed impossible.

Defeats that stayed longer than expected.

Players who arrived and left.

Rooms that no longer exist.

People who once watched from the chair beside them.

The adult knows that most matches will eventually blur into one another.

This one might too.

Or one touch may separate itself from everything around it.

That possibility is still enough.

The teams appear.

Conversation changes.

The lineup is checked one last time.

A message is sent.

Someone who had been thinking about something else ten minutes earlier is now watching the tunnel.

The child asks a question.

The adult answers.

Then both look toward the same screen.
Elsewhere, players gather on a neighborhood pitch.
One puts the ball down.
Another walks backward.
There are no stands.
No broadcast.
No thousands waiting.
Only a few people, some uneven grass, and a game about to begin.
The scale changes.
The waiting does not.
For a few seconds, nothing has happened.
The score is level.
No mistake has been made.
No chance has been missed.
No memory has been created yet.
Everything is still available.
The referee looks at the players.
A child edges closer to the television.
An adult settles into a familiar seat.
Someone in a café stops speaking halfway through a sentence.
Different places.
Different lives.
The same brief suspension.
Then the whistle sounds.
A player touches the ball.
And somewhere, almost immediately, someone leans forward.

About the Author

Moawiah Naffaa is a researcher and writer whose work and interests span medicine, neuroscience, human and artificial intelligence, meaning, and the biological processes that shape health and disease.

His scientific background has shaped the way he looks at ordinary human experiences—not only by asking what happens, but by asking what is happening beneath the surface: how attention shifts, how expectations form, how the body prepares before conscious thought catches up, how emotion changes memory, and how identity can alter the meaning of the same event.

When the Ball Moves grew from bringing that perspective to football.

The game offers an unusually vivid place to observe many of these processes at once. A supporter leans before a pass arrives. Thousands of strangers recognize danger almost together. One second survives in memory while much of a season disappears. A team of people we may never meet somehow becomes *we*.

Through football, Naffaa explores a larger question: **why events happening somewhere else can move so much inside us.**

His writing brings together scientific curiosity and the lived experience of everyday life, looking for the hidden processes beneath things that often feel too familiar to question.

www.ingramcontent.com/pod-product-compliance
Lightning Source LLC
LaVergne TN
LVHW010737061126
851857LV00014B/1517
* 9 7 9 8 2 5 6 2 9 8 2 9 6 *